MW01279864

# FORMERLY
# FLUFFY

## Been-There-Done-That
## Insights On Losing Weight
## Without Losing Your Mind

### Carrie Carlson

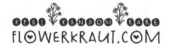

REAL RANDOM RARE
FLOWERKRAUT.COM

Cover design by
TimmDesign
timmdesign.work

ISBN (print) 978-1-7333565-0-3
ISBN (eBook) 978-1-7333565-1-0

# Dedication

For you. Yes, you. I wrote this for you.

# Contents

# INTRODUCTION
## This Book's for You

If you're the same brand of geek as me, the kind that reads all those pages in a book that come before the page numbered "1", you likely noticed that this book is dedicated to you. If you're not that brand of geek, it's dedicated to you as well, you just didn't read that page—and you're probably not reading this page either for that matter, it does have a roman numeral after all. I could have gone with my husband, my parents, my children, my sister, the friend who recommended the book and eating plan that got my weight loss process started… But, when I considered what led me to undertake this book project, it only seemed fitting that it should be dedicated to you. Don't worry, all those other people get their moment in the Acknowledgments section.

This book was born out of people like you asking me for been-there-done-that advice from my weight loss journey. I longed to be able to give them what I had learned, but time and lack of organization of my thoughts limited how much I could share. Ideally, I would love to be able to sit down one-on-one over coffee once a week with each person who asks and talk about it all as a couple of friends. But I don't like coffee and all of us are short on time. And, I needed to get some order to things. Lots of little tidbits were floating around in my head. Add to that my tendency to go down rabbit trails and extreme nervousness when having conversations with human beings, and you have a recipe for... SQUIRREL! See what I mean? What made me think that a shortage of time and a tendency toward attention deficit disorder would make writing a book more doable than one-on-one time is a great mystery to me.

I do know one thing; I've been where you are—firmly in Obese Class II, headed for Class III (a.k.a. morbid obesity), and beyond discouraged. You've had it with diets. Exercise leaves you feeling like you want that half-hour of your life back to do something you actually enjoy. And if you hear one more person who has a normal BMI, or even an overweight one, talk about how they need to lose 5 pounds, you'll scream. You'd give your eye teeth to be classified as just overweight. You're tired of being fluffy, but nothing seems to work. You have little hope and are one step away from refusing to try yet another approach you are just going to fail at. Been there, done that. In fact, I had gotten to the point that I did refuse to try anything. I was done.

So, this book's for you. Grab a cup of coffee (none for me, thanks) and let's talk.

One final thing to note before we get going. My advice is just that, my advice. It is knowledge and insight from *my* experience. The diet, nutrition, and fitness information presented here should not be your sole source of information, nor is it a substitute for the advice and care of your physician.

When making any changes to your diet, nutrition, or fitness habits, consult with your physician to determine what is appropriate for your individual circumstances.

# CHAPTER 1
# Honesty is The Best Policy

I feel like the first sentence of this book should be, "I've struggled with my weight all my life." After more than three years of hearing weight loss testimonies, they all seem to start out that way. And maybe mine should too, but not in the way this phrase usually implies. For most stories that start that way, it is code for, "I was overweight as a child and have been yo-yo dieting since my teens. It has left me feeling like a failure, with low self-esteem and depression for as long as I can remember." I, on the other hand, was a skinny child. Not underweight but thin enough that my mom describes her discovery of "slim" pants for girls as a godsend. And my leotard and tights for ballet class weren't exactly tight. But to say my weight was a struggle would be an overstatement. Other kids did not tease me about my weight, or lack thereof (though they did tease me about plenty of other things). I didn't feel insecure because of it. It's just the way I was.

To say I was obsessed with my weight as a teen would also be an overstatement. Like all good teen girls, I thought I should be thinner, and that if I could lose five or ten pounds, I

1

would be happier and have more friends. But overall, I was lazy, so dieting and exercise were relegated to three days here and there—not anything remotely close to obsession. This was a pattern that continued well into my twenties. And then I had babies.

Don't get me wrong. My children are what I consider my life's crowning achievement. I have put the last nineteen years into them and so far, by the grace of God, have ended up with three respectable human beings. I do not blame them for my weight gain, but my choices during pregnancy didn't do me any favors. To stave off morning sickness, I ate a lot of refined, processed carbs and didn't exercise any more than taking the dog for a quick once around the block. And, during my second and third pregnancies, preterm labor had me on modified bedrest for months. I gained close to 50 pounds with each pregnancy and 20 of it never left after each baby. By the time I was 35, I weighed 60 pounds more than I had when I graduated from college.

For about six months between my second and third babies, I tried the South Beach Diet® and joined a gym. The goal was to lose 40-50 pounds before getting pregnant again. I was determined. Or as determined as I get anyway. When the going gets tough, I tend to fold like a house of cards. With two children under the age of three, learning a new way of eating and getting to the gym felt like scaling Mount Everest. Motivation and energy to cook were nonexistent. Frozen burritos and macaroni & cheese from a box were about all I could manage, and they are not part of South Beach. The gym claimed it had childcare included in its membership. And it did...sort of...if they could keep a childcare provider employed and if that person actually showed up. In that six months' time, I lost about ten pounds and didn't look any different. It seemed like a lot of work for such little in the way of results. I gave up, figuring that once we were done having kids I'd deal with the weight.

So, for the next seven years, aside from the months I was pregnant, my weight hovered in the mid-180s to low-190s. My health numbers were poor for someone my age. Total cholesterol was nearing the warning level of 200; LDL ("bad" cholesterol) was 130, significantly over the high end of the normal range; and HDL ("good" cholesterol) was too low. My fasting blood sugar was dangerously close to 100, the level where a diagnosis of prediabetes is made. My blood pressure looked okay at the textbook 120/80. But, when you consider that my pre-fluffy normal blood pressure was more like 110/65, textbook was actually high for me. Additionally, I was diagnosed with obstructive sleep apnea and put on CPAP. The picture of health, I was not.

Family history wasn't on my side either. In the spring of 2009 my dad, at the age of 61, underwent quadruple bypass surgery following a "silent" heart attack. Given his personal and hereditary history the term silent is really not appropriate. For as long as I can remember, he has battled high blood pressure and hyperlipidemia—a.k.a. high cholesterol. His father, my grandfather, suffered his first stroke when my dad was still in high school and passed away at 68.

**In my mind, my fate was sealed.** I stood next to my dad's coronary intensive care hospital bed, when he was fresh out of post-op and on a ventilator, and stared at my future. I still could not manage to do anything about it.

And then I received a health surprise. For years, I had suspected I had hypothyroidism—underactive thyroid—and that it would explain the weight. Given a strong family history on both sides of thyroid disorders, both overactive and underactive, this was not unlikely. I pursued it with a couple of doctors only to be told my thyroid was fine. However, shortly after my diagnosis of sleep apnea, I woke up one morning and noticed my left eye felt like there was an eyelash in it. Upon investigation, in an attempt to remove the offending eyelash, I discovered that my left eye was bulging. I didn't have an eyelash in my eye at all. My eyeball was protruding so far that my lashes were brushing it when I blinked. It was also being pushed so far forward that my lashes touched the lens of my glasses. I immediately made an appointment with my doctor. Five doctors later, it was discovered that I had a form of hyperthyroidism—overactive thyroid—known as Grave's Disease. Grave's Disease is an autoimmune disorder that causes the body to start attacking itself, often causing unexplained weight loss. Mine was a form known as Grave's ophthalmopathy. In this form, thyroid antibodies cause the body to attack the muscles and tissues of only one eye, not both as is often the case with standard Grave's Disease. This was causing proptosis—bulging of the eye. The fix? Turns out there isn't one. Because, in my case, the levels of thyroid hormones in my blood were normal, supplementing them with artificial hormones wasn't called for. There was nothing else to do but wait for it to run its course. And in the meantime, you take prednisone to prevent it from getting worse. One of the more notorious side effects of prednisone is weight gain. Over the course of two years on periodic courses of prednisone I gained another 30-ish pounds. Since the alternative was potential loss of vision in my left eye due to swelling compromising the optic nerve, it was a small price to pay in the overall scheme of things.

Seeing the scale surpass 200 pounds in a non-pregnant state though was heartbreaking all the same.

On top of these things that all seemed stacked against me, I have suffered from anxiety and depression since at least my tweens and have been taking medication for it since I was in my mid-20s. Barring a miracle, I will never not have to take medication for it. For me, the roots of it are biochemical and medication is necessary. As is the case with many medications, particularly mental health ones, weight gain is a possible side effect of those I take. I don't think they had a significant impact on my weight gain. I took them all throughout my weight loss journey, and still take them, with no weight gain problems. However, the anxiety and depression themselves were exacerbated by the excess weight in three ways. First, looking in the mirror, at the scale, or at the size of my clothing left me feeling horrible about myself. Despite all the positive self-esteem education in school systems and self-help articles in women's magazines, we still live in a culture where beauty reigns and thinness is prized. Experts can preach, "Size doesn't matter," and "Love yourself as you are," all they want, but when what you see being valued by others is thin and flawless it is hard to swallow the psychobabble. And, being obese meant I had little energy or desire to exercise. Regular physical exercise is important to mental health. But I was in a catch-22 of no energy to exercise that then led to further depression meaning even less energy for exercise. Finally, it all—family history, medical diagnoses, no energy, having to learn better food choices— seemed so impossible to overcome, which fueled even more despair. This led to emotional eating that packed on more pounds. It was all so hopeless. I was defeated and believed that if God wanted me skinny, He would have made me that way. It was going to take a miracle because I couldn't do it myself. Little did I know that God did have plans to make me skinny again, but not in the way I figured a miracle would happen. I envisioned the miracle as something along the lines of waking up one morning and just being 100 pounds lighter. Instead, it started in the form of a book via a person I didn't even know yet.

I can hear what you're thinking right now, "Tell me what the book was. Give me the list of what you did so I can follow it." You might even be thumbing through the rest of this book looking for the name of the book that got me started or the list of checkboxes and recipes—spoiler alert, they aren't here (but please don't stop reading, there is something here that is just as, and possibly even more, important). We'll get to the name of the book in a little bit but, as you'll see, it's really not important. First, though, I need to give you some ground rules for reading the rest of my story.

## What This Book Won't Give You

There are four things this book won't give you:

1. The best diet to follow
2. A quick fix for obesity
3. A magic formula to follow to lose weight
4. Guarantees of almost any kind, except as noted in the What This Book Will Give You section below

The reason for this is simple, there is no best diet, quick fix, magic formula, or guarantees for anything (except death and taxes). And, anyone who tells you there are is lying or seriously delusional. They likely have something to gain, particularly financially, from convincing you there are. I realize this may be disappointing, or even heartbreaking, for you and you're giving yourself (and me) a good under-your-breath muttering about having wasted good money on this book. So, I'll repeat my earlier plea, please don't stop reading. There is something here that can benefit you. I believe that with all my heart. Not because I am some great weight loss motivator. Lord knows, the last thing I am is a cheerleader. I can't take classes at the gym because I'd be tempted to deck the trainer/coach the first time she said, "KEEP GOING, LADIES! ONLY FIVE MORE!" But I do truly believe that humans are allowed to experience things so they can help others.

## What This Book Will Give You

So, if I can't give you the best diet to follow, a quick fix, a magic formula, or any guarantees, what can I give you? The four things I can give you are:

1. Honesty - I don't know about you, but I'm fed up with elephants in the corner. You know, those things we all know are issues but no one wants to talk about—things that are embarrassing, might offend someone, or would require us to have to take a hard look at our own behavior if they are addressed. At times my honesty may seem brutal. Stay with me. My intention is to help, not hurt. I won't say it if I don't think it can benefit someone. See my challenge for you below.

2. Insight - Believe me when I say I guarantee I have had to take hard looks at my behavior on every issue in this book. This is the only guarantee I can make. I am giving you the insights I have had as a result. It's been-there-done-that experience. Not

everyone will experience the same things, but there are lessons to learn just the same.

3. Hope - You are not alone. It is not hopeless. That's as cheerleader as I get. My goal is to provide hope by providing honesty and insight.

4. Sanity - A weight loss journey can quickly spiral out of control psychologically. Is it worth exchanging a sound mind for a better-looking body? I don't believe so. And I don't think you really do either. I know what it's like to be so unhappy and miserable in your own body that, at first glance, it seems desirable to trade anything to feel better about what you see in the mirror. In the end though, such a trade will just leave you a different kind of miserable. There is a better way.

## My Challenge To You

Be honest with yourself. When you're offended don't retreat. Instead, ask yourself why you are reacting that way. Notice I didn't say, "*If* you're offended." There are bound to be things I say that will hit a nerve for you. I'm going to share a lot of things that hit a nerve for me the first time I encountered them. Our human reaction, when confronted with things that make us uncomfortable, is to run and hide, all the while covering our ears and shouting, "La, la, la, can't hear you!" Or worse, we become angry and lash out at the messenger, claiming they don't know what they are talking about or accusing them of being mean and uncaring. However, something provoking a strong reaction is doing so for a reason. Stop, take a couple of deep breaths, and ask yourself why it is giving you a case of the porcupines—what we call it in our house when someone is getting all upset and bristly. If you do, you may find there

FORMERLY FLUFFY

is something you need to deal with. It may even be so big of an issue for you that professional help is warranted. Or you may find that, upon reflection, your reaction was knee-jerk, and it really isn't that big of a deal for you. But you won't know which of those is the case unless you are willing to honestly explore it.

9

# CHAPTER 2
# **Why Diets Fail**

Let's take a minute here to clear up the term diet. Because the word has two meanings and this is a book about weight loss, this is a bit tricky. Diet can refer, in a general sense, to what one eats. More often, in our Western, weight-obsessed culture, the word diet is used to refer to a temporary way of eating designed to result in weight loss. I tend to use the word both ways and leave it to context to indicate which I'm meaning.

It turns out I had plenty of company in my quest to lose weight. At any given time, up to half of all Americans say they are trying to lose weight. Half. That's a lot of people—somewhere in the neighborhood of 45 million. How many actually succeed? It's hard to tell. A popular, but unverifiable statistic, is that 95% of dieters fail. An article in the *American Journal of Public Health* concludes that within any given year a mere 1 in 7 obese women and 1 in 8 obese men will be successful in achieving a 5% weight loss. And, there is only a 1 in 124 chance for those women and a 1 in 210 chance for the men to drop enough weight to be considered a "normal" weight. Maintaining weight loss success has equally dismal statistics. Within five years, at least one- to two-thirds of those who lose weight will have gained the weight back, and often a few more pounds as well.[1] For those of us who need to shed pounds, these numbers are not encouraging.

On the surface, losing weight is not rocket science—or even brain surgery.

Broken down to the basics, one loses weight by consuming fewer calories than one burns. Not hard to understand. The actual biology is a little more complicated and many theories are out there about how to accomplish this deficit. But the bottom line really is that simple. If it's so simple, then how come so many people are unsuccessful at weight reduction?

There are two main ways to accomplish a calorie deficit conducive to weight loss. One is to eat enough to be satisfied and have slightly fewer calories than you need to make it 3-4 hours before you eat again. That way, your body has to use it all for survival and use a little bit of what is stored too. The second method is known as intermittent fasting. Various formulas for intermittent fasting exist, but all of them operate on the premise that you eat normally for a period of time and then completely fast for a period of time, consuming nothing except water/calorie-free beverages during the fast. The two most popular ways to do this are 16:8 or 5:2. When using the 16:8 ratio, you eat normally 8 hours per day and fast for the remaining 16 hours. In 5:2, you eat normally 5 days per week and fast for 2 days. The key in each method is fasting long enough that your body has no choice but to use its stored energy. When and how much you eat are only part of the problem, however.

## Carbs: Friend or Foe? Actually Both

Just a calorie deficit at the end of the day isn't going to allow you to lose weight. Here's why. Most of us consume what is referred to as the standard American diet (SAD) or Western pattern diet (WPD). The hallmark of SAD/WPD is high consumption of refined, processed carbohydrates; white potatoes; sugar; corn; corn syrup, including high-fructose corn syrup; and high-sugar drinks. These foods all wreak havoc on blood sugar, which leads to fat storage.

We're constantly bombarded with, "Eat fewer refined/simple carbohydrates," and "We consume too much sugar." So let me just take a minute to explain what sugar and refined/simple carbs are, how they work in your body, and why not all carbs are minions of Satan. Understanding this concept was a huge eye-opener for me, which is why I'm explaining it here. Just a caveat, this explanation will be VERY simple—like kindergarten simple. The actual process in the body is quite complex and involves several hormones. I'm purposely keeping it simple because you don't need to know the names of all the hormones, where they act, and what they do exactly to get the point of why simple carbs and sugars are not your friends.

First, let me define simple carbohydrates and sugar. Simple carbs are high glycemic index (GI) foods. Anything made with standard, everyday white or wheat flour falls into this category. Products such as bread, tortillas, pitas, pasta, cakes, donuts, bars, etc. are all comprised largely of simple carbohydrates. White rice, white potatoes, carrots, and corn are also high glycemic carbs. Sugar is the obvious white granulated sugar, but sugar also includes brown sugar, molasses, agave, honey, fruit juice, corn syrup, high fructose corn syrup, fructose, dextrose, lactose, maltose, and sucrose, among others. The code for identifying sugar is looking for words ending in the suffix -ose. Not all -ose ending words are sugar, but the vast majority are. And don't be fooled by the label "organic" in front of any of the names for sugar. The organic status of sugar does not change its blood sugar spiking characteristics. What exactly does this blood sugar spiking have to do with obesity?

Imagine a value meal from your favorite fast-food joint— a nice big, juicy burger (or chicken, if you must) on a bun with a medium fry and a medium soft drink. The meat is protein and fat. Any cheese involved is fat with a small amount of protein and a few carbs. The fries and bun are carbs—largely simple, high GI carbs. And if your soft drink is not diet, it's a simple, high GI carb as well. Most of the volume of the meal is high GI carbs. Like your mother taught you, you clean your plate because there are starving children in Africa. As those carbs hit your digestive system, they are broken down into and released as sugar into your bloodstream. Because they are high GI, simple carbs, your system doesn't have to do much work on them before sending the sugar right into your blood. This causes a rapid rise, or spike, in your blood sugar. But your body can't handle large amounts of sugar in the bloodstream for very long. If it doesn't do something about the increase in blood sugar, you will die. So, it releases insulin to clean up the sugar. Some sugar is used by your muscles, but because you've consumed way more than your muscles can use right at the moment, it has to do something with the leftovers. So, it packs the extra away by sending it to your fat cells to use at a later time. The meal also included some fat but, because your body was so busy using and cleaning up the sugar, it couldn't use the fat. The fat also had to go somewhere because it can't just sit there forever waiting. So, it took up residence around your organs and between your skin and muscles—for some reason, it has a particular affinity for the liver, abdomen, and thighs.

This storage of excess carbs/sugar as fat would not be a problem except for the fact that over the last hundred years or so we have become a more sedentary culture. Many of us no longer work in occupations that use all the energy we consumed at our last meal. We consume food in quantities far in excess of what we can use in the relatively short period of time we have between meals and snacks. Nowadays, by the time the body needs to go to those fat stores to use that energy reserve (roughly the 3-4 hour mark), we are eating again. Every time we eat we're giving it more carbs/sugar and fat, starting the whole process over before any stored energy gets used. So even if you eat less at your next meal, the damage has already been done with the stored fat from the previous meal. This is also why exercise isn't terribly effective at burning stored fat. By the time you get your workout in, you have stored the extra calories as fat, and your body isn't going to give that stored fat up readily.

That said, not all carbs are bad. Complex carbohydrates like those found in oatmeal, whole sprouted grains, beans/legumes, and vegetables are much lower on the glycemic index scale. They result in less drastic blood sugar swings than those caused by their simple, refined cousins. As the name **Not all carbs are bad.** complex suggests, your body has to do more work to break them down before sending their sugar into your bloodstream. This breaking down process leads to more of a slow, steady trickle of sugar into the blood, and this helps keep blood sugar from rising rapidly. Your body can use the slow trickle without having to go into a panic mode of insulin-fueled cleanup, thereby avoiding storing the excess sugar as fat.

Fruit is also a healthier source of carbs, as long as it is eaten in its whole, unprocessed form. Because fruit contains significant simple sugars in its juice, it is important to consume fruit whole so you get the moderating factor of the fiber to prevent spiking blood sugar. Drinking fruit juice alone has a similar effect on blood sugar levels as eating a candy bar does. And canned fruit often has added syrup, so it is best to steer clear of that as well.

Hopefully, that helps clear up why carbohydrates have gotten a bad rap and how they can still have a place in your diet. Cut back on the simple, refined, high glycemic index carbs—what I often refer to as "the white stuff"—and include plenty of vegetables with reasonable amounts of other healthy complex carbs. Your body will thank you.

## I Think, Therefore I Am

Weight loss is largely a mental issue. In a sense, it could be argued that it is possible to think yourself thin. Don't take that to mean I am promoting some New Age philosophy that the mind creates reality. You can't just sit on the sofa eating bon-bons repeating, "I am skinny," and expect to have the body of a supermodel in a few weeks or months or, well, ever. However, the thought patterns of the mind do play a big role, possibly as big as diet and exercise themselves, in how successful your journey will be. What is often the biggest mental problem with weight loss is that we grasp at straws trying to find the answer to our weight problem in the form of externals, like what and how much we exercise. Those answers always come up empty because nothing about us changes—not our hearts, not our minds, not our habits. The reason these things don't change is the failure to get real with ourselves about some very key things.

## Self-Deception

We lie to ourselves all the time. I have heard it suggested that self-deception may be necessary to a degree to keep us sane. That knowing the whole truth about ourselves and the world around us would land us in the looney bin. And there may be some truth to this idea, particularly if one does not have some kind of faith in a higher power. But how does this self-deception play out in weight loss? The major way we deceive ourselves is by fooling ourselves into thinking we are adhering to a diet when we really aren't. It is critical to follow the eating plan you choose all the time, particularly when starting on the journey. Only doing it 80% of the time is not really doing it, it's dabbling in it. Just having read about a plan and understanding (and even believing in) the concepts is not doing it. So, the first thing to ask yourself is, "How closely am I really following the plan?" Then give yourself an honest answer. If your answer sounds something like, "Well…I mostly…" or "I stick to it for meals but snacks…" then you are unearthing deception. The other area of weight loss where self-deception often shows up is in how much we're eating. We tend to underestimate the quantity of food we consume. Sometimes this is deliberate because we feel too ashamed to admit we eat a pint of ice cream at one time. Other times, it is unconscious because we graze or snack without realizing it or we just don't recognize what reasonable serving sizes look like. It's hard to be honest with ourselves. Believe me, I know. But once you can be honest with yourself, you can change the behaviors inhibiting your progress.

## Losing Weight Isn't Going to Make You Happy

I don't know how to make that statement gently. Too many of us have bought into the lie that being thinner is going to make us happy. Technically, I suppose, this would fall under self-deception because it's a lie we've been fed (no pun intended) for so many years by movies, television, music, books, and even friends and family that we've internalized it and now tell it to ourselves. The truth is, losing weight is just going to make you a smaller version of you. So, if you're a miserable overweight person, you'll likely be a miserable skinny person. Yes, weight loss can help alleviate depression, anxiety, and other issues, but it will not make them go away completely. Losing weight isn't going to make life all sunshine and roses. Skinny people suffer from the same things the rest of us do. Spend some time thinking about why you want to lose weight. As always, be honest. The socially acceptable answer is "to be healthier," but is that really the answer for you? Or is your answer something that is more along the lines of "to be more popular" or "so I'm not disgusted by what I see in the mirror"? Those are not wrong answers, but it is important to know what your motivations are and how likely losing weight is to be the fix. Part of your weight loss journey will need to involve making mental shifts. Depending on what your issues are, they may require you to seek the services of a mental health professional for help in dealing with them.

## "You"nique

"You do you," is the mantra of the day these days. Want purple hair? Go for it! Don't like what I am wearing? Hey, you do you. But as much as we talk about being ourselves, not comparing ourselves to others, and not conforming to the expectations of society, deep down human nature just seems to crave sameness.

The truth is, you are you. You are not me. You are not your neighbor. Or your best friend. Or your sister. Or the celebrity you see selling weight loss plans on TV. In a culture that so heavily embraces individuality, it seems that stating such a thing is eye-roll worthy. Yet for some reason, we believe that doing exactly the same things people we admire do will give us the exact same admirable qualities. When it comes to weight loss and almost anything else in life, there are so many variables that doing exactly what someone else has done does not guarantee getting the exact same results. Recognizing this uniqueness and leveraging it can make all the difference in your weight loss journey.

## Weight Loss Speed

Command-Z, a.k.a. Undo, has made life frustrating for me, as has having an ESC key. I have become so accustomed to being able to instantly undo my last computer actions, or escape out of processes I didn't mean to start, at the press of a button that when I encounter things that take longer to reverse (or worse, can't be reversed at all) I want to lay down kicking like a two-year-old and scream, "I WANT IT NOW!" It's the simultaneous blessing and curse of living in the Western world. Unfortunately, weight loss is one of those things that takes time. There is no command-Z or ESC key to undo weight gain. Weight loss can't be made instantaneous—oh, how I wish it could. And, how fast the loss happens varies from one person to another. Some will lose quite rapidly, particularly if they are coming from very poor eating habits. Others will feel like they are having a tug-of-war with every last extra ounce they want to send packing. Keep in mind, no one should lose more than 1-2 pounds per week. I know that sounds like a horribly slow rate, especially if you're in the position I was of needing to lose more than 50 pounds. But, to keep your loss healthy and sustainable, that's as fast as it should go. And, you didn't put the weight on at any faster rate than that, or even at that rate. If you had, you would have gained somewhere between 50 and 100 pounds in a year. So don't expect to take it off any faster.

## Body Type

No two bodies are the same. They come in all shapes and sizes. And, we usually want a shape and size we were not born with. Height, skeletal structure, genetics, metabolism, and a myriad of other factors influence how the same weight will look on different people. It is important to do some investigation on body type and identify what type you are to help prevent unrealistic expectations and goals.

Ectomorph, mesomorph, and endomorph. No, these are not three aliens from a science-fiction galaxy far, far away. These are the formal names of the three main body types. Ectomorphs are long and lean. They don't put on weight very easily, either in the form of muscle or body fat. Mesomorphs tend to have high metabolisms and are muscular. They put on muscle mass easily. Endomorphs have a tendency to store body fat and often appear pear-shaped. However, if you take a quick look around, or even just in the mirror, it quickly becomes obvious that three body types are woefully limited in describing most people—especially women. This limitation has led some diet and fitness coaches to develop other body type descriptions. Rectangle, triangle, inverted triangle, hourglass, round, oval, apple, pear—they start to sound like a geometry lesson with fruit salad thrown in. Fitness guru Teresa Tapp uses the terms long torso/short torso and long leg/short leg.[2] It doesn't matter which naming system you pick, the critical thing is to realize what shape you are and how it will determine what you can and can't expect to look like.

## Food Issues

We all have food issues, and like body type, our food issues are unique to each of us. Knowing your personal food issues, good and bad, is essential to transforming your diet into a healthier version to meet weight loss goals and live with long term. Do you like sweets? Are you a grazer or a meal eater or both? What kinds of carbohydrates do you prefer—sweet treats and baked goods or bread or pasta? Do you tend toward extremes—binge eating or food restriction? Do you medicate emotions with food? Grab a piece of paper and a pen. Take an honest inventory of your positive and negative food habits and write them down. This is more than making a list of things you need to give up or change. Even something like "I love kale," needs to go on the list. This list will be a vehicle to help you evaluate what eating plan will be most doable for you. It will help you plan for success by knowing what your relationship is to food. Don't spend too much time analyzing the items on your list as "good" or "bad." This isn't an exercise in beating yourself up or boasting. We're just stating facts. You may find that you uncover things you need professional help with, like eating disorders—which, by the way, doesn't only mean anorexia or bulimia. Any persistent eating behavior that negatively impacts physical and/or emotional health is an eating disorder. Don't be afraid to get help, and don't berate yourself for having the issue and needing help. That won't get you anywhere. Start with the following list of food preference statements, but additional items may come to mind as you go. Put them all on your list.

- ∂ I prefer to eat sweet things like candy bars, cake, cookies, donuts, etc. rather than savory or salty foods.
- ∂ You can keep the sweets, give me things like cheese and meat.
- ∂ I like to have a bedtime snack every night.
- ∂ I do not eat breakfast.
- ∂ I enjoy/detest eating vegetables.
- ∂ I love/hate fruit.
- ∂ I feel it is important to track every calorie I take in.
- ∂ I have no clue how many calories I eat in one day.
- ∂ I do not like to drink plain water.
- ∂ I'm a "carbivore"—I love pasta, bread, potatoes, baked goods, etc.
- ∂ I prefer eating out to home-cooked meals.
- ∂ I refuse to give up the following foods:
  _____
- ∂ When I was growing up, my food choices were controlled or criticized by others.
- ∂ I prefer to eat small amounts of food throughout the day rather than big meals.
- ∂ I often forget or am too busy to eat.
- ∂ I regularly overeat.
- ∂ I drink regular (non-diet) soda all day.
- ∂ I drink diet soda all day.
- ∂ I like to have dessert after meals.
- ∂ I do not like the following foods:
  _____
- ∂ I eat when I'm upset/anxious/happy/bored/etc.

∂   I eat at the same set times every day.

∂   When I was growing up, we regularly went without food or did not have enough food due to economic or parental neglect circumstances.

∂   I love/hate to cook.

∂   I love/hate to bake.

∂   I like salty, crunchy snacks like potato chips and popcorn.

∂   I drink coffee all day (straight black or with minimal cream/sugar).

∂   I drink water all day.

∂   I drink coffee-based drinks (i.e. lattes, cappuccinos, macchiatos, etc.).

∂   I go out to eat with friends often.

∂   I regularly eat meals with extended family.

∂   I eat at one or more special occasions (i.e. birthdays, anniversaries, holidays, etc.) per month.

∂   I drink alcohol regularly.

∂   Chocolate. (Need I say more?)


Once you have made your list, you're ready to start looking for a new way of eating that will work for you.

# CHAPTER 3
# **The Best Diet**

I wish I could ask everyone who turned to this chapter without completely reading the Introduction and first two chapters to send me a dollar. After all, this one looks like it would contain what you and ultimately what we all want—to cut to the chase and find the magic formula. If you haven't read chapters 1 and 2 completely, please go back and do so before continuing. Consider reading the Introduction as well. They're short, and this chapter isn't going anywhere.

Now that you're back…

Late in 2014, my family relocated. In terms of distance, it wasn't a huge move. But, it was significant enough that I had to make new friends, get new doctors, and develop new routines. I was going through a period of mourning as part of this transition when, at church one Sunday morning, I noticed an announcement for a women's Bible study starting that week. Studying Scripture is one of my favorite things to do, and it would be a good way for me to meet other women at our new church. So I signed up. With flashbacks of other instances of trying to join small groups, I was terrified, but I had to start somewhere. Little did I know how life-changing this group would be for me.

The topic of diets came up at some point in our weekly pre-study chit-chat, and one of the members mentioned she followed a plan called Trim Healthy Mama (THM). She had lost 20 pounds or so on it. I tuned out. Diets weren't for me. I had a whole lot more than 20 pounds to lose. And, if it was like any other diet, losing 5, 10, or even 20 pounds would be easy, and then it would stop working. I'd gain it all back plus. Why try something you are only going to fail at? I had dug in my heels. If I was going to be skinny, it was going to be an act of God.

Well, it kept popping up. Not every week and certainly not because my friend was trying to proselytize the rest of us food heathens, but another group member was trying it and would ask questions occasionally. Then one day, the *Trim Healthy Mama Plan* and *Trim Healthy Mama Cookbook* somehow ended up in my cart at Amazon. You know how it is. You're at Amazon getting a few things you need, and you ask yourself, "Is there anything not really expensive but also not a necessity I can just throw in this order to make getting a box full of aquarium filters and printer toner fun?" Please tell me I'm not the only one who does this. The books arrived, and I set them on my footstool—for months. I still wasn't sure I was going to use them. But unread books drive me nuts. After a couple months, I *had* to read the plan book because I couldn't own a book that I hadn't read, not because I actually planned on doing what it said. I was just weeks away from turning 42. As I read, a couple of weird things happened. First, it made sense. Second, I thought I might actually be able to do it—not lose the weight per se but follow the THM way of eating for more than a few days. And finally, just sitting there reading about it, I swear I could feel myself shrinking. There is no possible way that could have been true, short of that miracle I said it would take to get me to lose weight, but I felt a strange sensation all the same. Rest assured, I wasn't really shrinking at that point. Days before my birthday, I had my annual physical. I weighed 225 pounds, my heaviest ever. Three days after my 42nd birthday, I started THM. I didn't have a debate with myself about it. I didn't get all hyped saying, "I'm going to lose this weight!" It was more like walking into a dark room and flipping the light switch. I didn't think, "It's dark in here I should turn a light on." I just reached for the switch and flipped it. The thing is, I didn't even really believe it would work. I grew up in the low-fat '80s. There was no way a diet that didn't ban red meat and cheese, severely limit calories, and said eat until you're satisfied could actually work. So, I set up a science experiment. For one year, I would eat the THM way. I would track my weight, measurements, lipid profile numbers[*], blood pressure, and fasting blood sugar. That way, I could say I had given it an honest effort, and it turned out to be just another diet gimmick. I would like to note here, I'm using the term science experiment loosely. I'm very aware it wasn't really a *scientific* experiment. Lack of a control group, double-blindness, etc. disqualifies it from being truly a science experiment, but at least I would be able to say I had proved it wouldn't work for me. We'll get to what happened later. First, there are three truths about diets we need to get out in the open.

---

[*] total cholesterol, HDL, LDL, VLDL, and triglycerides

#1 There is no best diet for weight loss.

I said it before, and I'll say it again. There is no best diet, quick fix, magic formula, pill, powder, or shake that is going to work for everyone. If there were a best diet, quick fix, or magic formula that worked for everyone, we'd all know about it and use it. We know that. But the lure of quick, easy, and painless is so powerful that we are willing to set aside common sense on the outside chance the latest fad is true. This is also absurd when you really think about it. If the latest fad turns out to be truly a quick, easy, painless cure for obesity, are you really going to miss out on it? Something like that would be big news, taking the world by storm. It wouldn't disappear, never to be available again. Here's the truth: The diet/weight loss business is a $70 *billion* per year industry.[3] That's a ton of money, and a lot of people are more than willing to do whatever they can to get their hands on a share of it, including telling you they have the secret cure to the weight loss woes.

On top of that, everyone who loses weight thinks the diet they follow is the best. Keto people believe keto is the way to go. Paleo people say paleo is the best. "Mamas," as those who follow THM call themselves, think their way is best. Those who lose on Weight Watchers™, now known as WW™, or NutriSystem® are all about those plans. It's a human nature thing. We believe that about almost anything we do. If it works for me, it must be the best way. But, due to the infinite variety of humans, almost anything works for at least some people. Weight loss is no different. Most diet plans will work for at least some people for at least awhile. The trick is to find the plan that works for you and that you can follow for the rest of your life.

## #2 You're going to have to think.

The thing is, most people don't want to think. They want a pill, powder, or shake that will allow them to eat whatever they want at the moment and have the model-thin body the media brainwashes us into thinking is the ideal body. They want something that will tell them what to eat, how much of it to eat, and when to eat it like some magic formula. But eventually, they get tired of that and go back to their old habits because it is too restrictive. If you want freedom, you have to be willing to engage your brain. When children are young, parents don't give them much freedom. Mom and dad decide when they will go to bed, what they will eat, when they need to nap, and where they are allowed to go alone. As they get older, their parents allow them more freedom because, as they grow, they are capable of higher-level thought processes allowing them to make wise choices on their own. People who refuse to think cannot be free because, like small children, they will destroy themselves by making bad or even flat out dangerous decisions. Yes, at first whatever eating plan you decide to learn will seem like a lot of work, just like when you first learned how to read, but it does become second nature if you keep at it.

## #3 You're going to have to make lifelong changes.

Your diet (temporary) is going to have to become your diet for life (permanent). Stop thinking of it as a plan or diet and think of it as "the way I eat." You didn't think of your old way of eating as a plan or diet or burden. I found it helpful to think along the lines of "I don't eat pasta." Period. As if it were a fact just like the fact I don't eat peas or bananas because I don't like them. That way it never even crosses my mind to buy pasta just like I never even consider buying peas or bananas. To lose weight and sustain that loss, whatever way of eating you choose is going to need to focus on changing habits and be doable long-term. You can't follow a plan just long enough to lose the weight and then go back to eating the way you did before. When I said I would do THM for a year, I didn't impose that year with the intention to go back to my old ways. I imposed it as a limit to when I would conclusively say that THM did or didn't work for me. If it worked, I knew I was going to have to continue eating that way to sustain any loss. If it didn't work, I could say I had given it ample time. Then I could either try something else or, more likely, go back to eating the way I always had—and likely put on even more weight. The way you have always eaten is a major reason why you are overweight, meaning you're going to have to change the way you eat going forward to prevent going back to overweight. You have to decide how much you want it. You'll put your time, effort, and money into what's really important to you. And then you will need to accept new key principles as being "just the way I eat now."

## Finding Your Diet

How do you find the diet that will work for you and that is sustainable? This is where that list of food issues comes in. I did not make an issues list when I started out. It is something I have learned along the way. If I had made a list, it would have looked something like:

$\partial$   I am not willing to give up cheese or red meat.

$\partial$   I do not particularly crave sweets.

$\partial$   I do not like fruit.

$\partial$   I prefer to eat out and enjoy fast food.

$\partial$   I do not like to cook.

∂   I like salty and savory foods.

∂   I drink diet soda all day.

∂   I do not like to drink plain water.

∂   I'm not a big fan of chicken, especially white meat.

∂   I have no desire to count calories, macros, points, etc.

There are other things I could add, but you get the idea.

Once you have your list, start looking at various eating plans. There are tons of them, so you'll have to pick two or three to start with. Don't pay any attention to how many pounds, or how fast, they claim you will lose. Evaluate them against your list of issues. Using my list above as an example, any style of eating that required counting calories, macros, or points was not going to work for me so that would be the first thing I'd look for. If the plan had counting requirements, I would disqualify it right there. Now, counting might not be a deal-breaker for you. That's okay. This is just an example. From there, I'd look at the red meat and dairy restrictions. I'll eat chicken, but I don't want to eat it more than once a week. And I love cheese. That means I want to make sure red meat and cheese are allowed in more than occasional or garnish amounts. Because I don't drink plain water unless it is ICE cold, I need to drink something flavored to get my daily water requirements, making it important to select a plan that allowed, or had recipes for, drinks I could use to replace my diet soda habit. I eat out a lot and enjoy eating out more than eating at home. I needed something with principles I could use to eat tasty things at restaurants without eating things that were bad for me. Again, these are just examples particular to me for illustration. Your issues may be, and likely are, different. That's okay. The important thing is for you to evaluate potential plans against your list. You won't find a plan that will meet all of your criteria. That is the way you currently eat, and it has packed on the pounds. Let's face it, you will have to choose a way of eating that requires you to make adjustments and give up some stuff. The trick is to find the one that you are willing to say, "As long as I can _____, I don't mind giving up _____."

## Some General Guidelines
While I won't tell you what specific diet is the "best" for you to follow, I do want to offer some general things to look for in a healthy eating plan.

1. Look for a plan that focuses on eating low-glycemic foods. In general, this means it avoids added sugars, refined/processed carbohydrates, and other high-glycemic foods like white rice, white potatoes, carrots, fruit juices, corn, etc. Meals should focus on a protein source and use non-starchy vegetables as filler rather than potatoes, bread, pasta, rice, etc. That is not to say that high-glycemic foods are to never be eaten, but they must be used sparingly, which is not how they are present in the typical American/Western diet.

2. Avoid plans that have you purchase products such as prepackaged or prepared food, supplements, pills, powders, shakes, etc. The main reason to avoid those plans is those prepackaged and prepared foods are often highly processed and filled with stuff that gives them a fairly long shelf-life, usually in the form of sugars. The

other reason is this, a plan that requires you eat their food isn't interested in your long-term success but in their long-term bottom line. They are in it to make as much money as possible. Remember, there is $70 billion per year up for grabs here. And finally, if you are dependent on their products for success, what will you do when their products are no longer available? Some argue that Trim Healthy Mama is a plan requiring you to use their products, but it isn't. I don't *have* to purchase anything besides real, whole foods that I can get at my local grocery store to make THM work. I *can* purchase things like sweetener and flour substitutes from THM, but it is not required. There are sweeteners and flours readily available in most grocery stores that will work on the THM plan just fine.

3. Think very seriously before adopting a plan that involves counting things like calories or macros (protein, fats, carbohydrates). Remember, you are going to have to eat this way for a lifetime. Counting takes a lot of time, and many people who try it quickly get tired of having to do math every time they eat. Therefore, they give up—usually before they see much in the way of results. That said, a plan that involves counting may be something that works for your personal situation. I'm just advising you to honestly evaluate if that type of diet is a fit for the type of person you are. Do you really want to be counting things for every bite of food you eat for the rest of your life?

4. Keep a food log, but do not use an app. Get a small

notebook—one about the size of this book is perfect. Every time you eat something, write it down with an honest approximation of how much you ate. Write it down immediately. Don't wait, or you'll forget. At times, I found this alone discouraged me from eating. I didn't want to take the time to write it down. Lazy? Yes, but it kept me honest with my food intake. You won't have to keep a food log forever. When starting out though it is invaluable to keep you honest and help you spot habits that may be tripping you up. I kept one for the first two years of my journey, long enough to have made my new way of eating a habit.

Why don't I recommend an app? Food tracking apps are, in my honest opinion, a waste of time and effort. It takes a lot of time to enter food, portion sizes, and calorie counts. You should be spending that time enjoying your meal and the company of those you are eating with rather than recording data. And don't fall for the trap that you would enjoy your meal and company and record the info later. You'll forget. By the time you remember, you will only have a vague recollection of what and how much you ate. Additionally, the calorie and macro count information in apps may not be correct or will be missing. Many of the apps rely on users submitting info to the database for other users to tap into. It is impossible to know if the person entering the info for 1% cottage cheese entered the correct info. If there isn't any info entered, it will be up to you to figure out its nutrition info and enter it yourself, sucking up even more of your time. I would say an app is a good way to log food intake only if you find you have a problem with calorie abuse (more on this later) or are adopting a plan that involves counting calories or macros.

5.  I strongly discourage using drinks like shakes and smoothies, even healthy ones, as meal replacements or snacks. Here's why. First, eating is about more than the flavor of food. The entire eating process—from chewing to flavor to fullness—is an important part of feeling satisfied. Just sipping a shake that tastes like cheesecake isn't going to really satisfy your desire for cheesecake. Often, you'll end up eating something else to get the sensation of chewing and being full, meaning you've ingested a lot of additional calories. And second, the human mind tends to think things we drink are calorie-free even though they may not be. Shakes and smoothies contain significant calories. It's really easy to fool yourself into thinking it is okay to have a snack an hour after you've had a shake because your mind thinks the shake didn't really count. Stick to actual food that you have to chew.

6.  Find something healthy to sip all day—not soda (either regular or diet), sports drinks, shakes, or anything with sugar or fat added (like designer coffee drinks). Most health gurus would suggest water. Other things that work are tea (iced or hot) or flavored water—as long as the flavoring doesn't have sugar in it. If you select a tea as your primary hydration method, do some research to make sure it is safe in large quantities. Some teas can be dangerous or interact with certain medications when consuming more than a couple of cups per day. You can

also google the term "Trim Healthy Mama Sippers" for recipes. Even though I am not suggesting Trim Healthy Mama as the best diet for everyone to follow, THM sipper recipes would be appropriate for anyone to use. They are flavored but are not a significant source of calories and suitable for drinking throughout the day. Sipping all day helps curb appetite and keeps you hydrated. As ironic as it may seem, dehydration will actually make your scale number increase.

7. Watch out for myths and hype. There's a lot of pseudoscience out there, and some of it is very convincing, so let's look at it in more detail.

## Myths, Hype, and Documentaries

"Margarine is one molecule away from being plastic!" Back in the "old" days, you got an email inbox full of these things. But thanks to social media and blogs, nowadays it is easier than ever to spread myths, half-truths, and outright propaganda about everything, including food. As you begin evaluating eating plans to find one that will fit you, it is important that you watch carefully for these types of things.

Four statements I regularly see that just make me cringe are:

1. [Some food product] is one molecule away from [some horrible poison], or a variation on this such as [Some food product] is chemically similar to [some horrible poison] or [Some food product] is used in making [some inedible/toxic product].

2. [Such and such food or supplement] is natural, so it's safe.

3. If you can't read all the ingredients on the package, don't eat it.

4. Do your own research

Let me start by saying, many times I actually agree with the underlying conclusion—i.e. that one should eat foods as close to their natural state as possible or that a natural sweetener is better than an artificial one. My beef (no pun intended) with these statements is that they are not logically sound and make healthy eaters appear to be fanatic cult members.

## Chemical Similarity is Irrelevant

Using the logic that something is chemically similar to a known poison is not relevant or proof that it is bad. Water and hydrogen peroxide are chemically similar—$H_2O$ vs. HO. One I will drink and require it to live. The other, not a good idea to drink in large quantities. One molecule, or even one atom, difference can mean a lot in terms of safety. The oxygen we need to live is a molecule containing two oxygen atoms. Ozone, on the other hand, is a molecule containing three oxygen atoms. It is dangerous to breathe. So, even if margarine is one molecule away from plastic, that isn't a valid argument that it is bad for you. A more compelling argument about why you should avoid margarine is that it often contains high amounts of trans fat. Trans fats lower high-density lipoproteins (HDL, a.k.a. good cholesterol) and therefore increase the risk for heart disease.

## The Natural = Safe Fallacy

The justifications of "it's natural" and "it's plant-based" for foods or supplements being safe is not legitimate either. Many things that are natural or plant-based and are not safe: tomato leaves, rhubarb leaves, opium, hemlock, oleander, some varieties of mushrooms, poison ivy—just to name a few. The phrase "too much of a good thing" exists for a reason. Nothing is completely safe, and too much of anything can be harmful. So, let's see the "natural" label and its cousins for what they are, marketing hype.

## Supercalifragilisticexpialidocious

Another popular mantra in the healthy eating world is to refuse to consume anything that contains ingredients that you can't pronounce. And, on the surface, this is great advice. Once you think about this a little though, a small problem develops. Everything has multiple names or labels. Sodium chloride=table salt. Sodium bicarbonate=baking soda. Aspartame=Equal. Sucralose=Splenda. Dihydrogen monoxide. Sounds scary, right? You know it by another name, water. Things can be renamed according to their chemical makeup. Plants and animals are often referred to using Latin-based binomial nomenclature, turning broccoli into *Brassica oleracea* L. var. *botrytis* L. Just because a name for something is difficult to pronounce doesn't mean it is bad for you. Just because you can pronounce something doesn't mean it's good for you. I can pronounce antifreeze, but if I see it on the label of a food, I'm not going to eat it.

## Googling is Not Research

What seems to be the final defense of many people touting sensational food claims is, "Do your own research." This is often used when you are questioning the hype rather than just jumping on the bandwagon. "Do your own research," is a polite way of saying, "La la la! Can't hear you!" Proponents of sensational food sound bites don't even want to entertain the possibility they have fallen for a myth or propaganda. People say they have done their own research. What they have done is googled the topic, read a few blogs written by self-proclaimed experts, watched a "documentary", and decided to believe the information that agrees with the preconceived notion that led them to google the topic to begin with. That is not research; it is a form of confirmation bias—finding information to support what one already believes is true. Research is reading actual scientific, peer-reviewed studies about all sides of the topic. For every article that says something is okay, there is one saying it will kill you. And ultimately, the truth is probably somewhere in between.

Because there are "documentaries", blogs/websites, and research by "professionals" out there that are pretty convincing that various foods are going to kill us all, it's important to remember a couple of things when viewing any type of information. First, the internet and relatively cheap technology make it possible for anyone to make a "documentary" with a few thousand dollars. And, launching a website that looks pretty professional can be done with just a few mouse clicks. Health and nutrition "documentaries" and blogs are often produced by people or groups convinced anything not grown organically by oneself, or that has been processed at all, is dangerous and the end of civilization. Additionally, blogging has increasingly become a way of making a living for many people. They earn a living by readers clicking on affiliate links or ads on their website. That doesn't necessarily mean they are publishing incorrect information, but it should cause one to think carefully about what they are reading. Is it possible for the author to be objective about the topic if you clicking a link in their blog will increase their paycheck?

Second, research and statistics can be manipulated. Research is often funded by companies with a vested interest in research turning out a certain way—making them or their product/cause look good or making a competitor/opposing cause look bad. In our modern world, this is typically accomplished "under the table" with seemingly unrelated transactions. Government agencies, universities, and research firms are often paid by companies in the form of grants, donations, or other lobby influences. But in the not so distant past, as recently as 55 years ago, the sugar industry flat-out bribed researchers to skew results to downplay the role of sugar in the development of heart disease and cast the blame on fat.[4]

Finally, research often merely shows an association between two or more things, but the mass media reports it as if causation has been established. It is important to verify what you are reading or hearing. Do research, but also think critically. Don't just look for the sound bites that agree with what you already believe. You haven't made an informed opinion unless you've seriously looked at all sides of an issue without bias.

Eating in response to the stresses of life and making food choices based on "margarine is one molecule away from plastic" hype are both forms of food bondage known as emotional eating. Emotional eating occurs when we self-medicate by overeating, not eating, or eating the wrong things to deal with or celebrate life events such as death, divorce, job stress, marriage trouble, money trouble, sadness, frustration, and joy. Another very valid area of emotional eating is making food decisions based on fads, hype, sound bites, and junk science. It is important to weigh statements about food safety and selection with a logical, not emotional, mind. Evaluating food safety from an emotional point of view allows you to be easily swayed when the next fad or hype headline comes along. It can also cause you to easily give up your healthier ways because you don't really understand or believe the why behind the information. Looking at the whole picture of a particular food will allow you to make a reasonable choice about its place in your diet.

## Cheating

No discussion of diet would be complete without taking a minute to talk about cheating. It seems as soon as you select a diet plan and make it past day three, all you can think about are the things that you're not allowed to eat and how badly you suddenly want to eat them. So, you say, "I'm just going to cheat a little and have a bite." Suddenly that one bite turns into a whole cake and days or weeks (or even months or years) of going back to old eating habits. It's yo-yo dieting, and we all know it doesn't work. This is why it is so important to know your food issues and carefully select an eating plan that you can turn into your new way of everyday eating—and why it's so important to be honest with yourself about how much you are truly following your chosen plan. It's easy to say, "I'm doing a keto diet," but be doing things like having fries with lunch every day because "a few won't hurt." Then you wonder why you're not losing weight and blame the diet saying, "Keto didn't work for me." My octogenarian father-in-law has been diagnosed with type 2 diabetes. He loves to tell us his home health nurse says he can eat whatever he wants "in moderation." And I don't doubt that is indeed what his nurse says. However, it's really easy to moderate yourself right out of moderation. Moderation of five different things adds up to not moderation. So how do you find balance? Here are a few tips:

## List your deal breaker foods.

For most people, there are no foods you have to completely cut out of your diet no matter what plan you follow. I realize this is somewhat controversial advice. All kinds of dieting camps promote cutting various foods. The current popular trend is to ban carbs and make protein a priority. Ketogenic diets focus on keeping carbs very low. Paleo diets avoid sugar, dairy, legumes, and grains. Even the THM plan I follow eliminates added sugar and encourages avoidance of high-glycemic foods in weight loss mode. I won't go into the reasons why these practices may be good, bad, or otherwise. But, as I mentioned, the SAD/WPD diet contains added sugars (added sugar is in nearly EVERYTHING; don't believe me, check the ingredients list of your container of table salt—dextrose will be listed—yes, there is sugar in salt), refined/processed carbohydrates, and high-glycemic foods like corn, white potatoes, and white flour in excessive amounts, so it is wise to limit consumption. It's okay to select a plan that limits some things but always maintain perspective. The trick is that you can't eat those things on a regular basis as part of your everyday meals. They can still be treats from time to time—once a month, three times a year, once a year—how often depends on the individual. If I select a plan that says, "You can never eat macaroni and cheese," and I really want macaroni and cheese, I would feel imprisoned by and angry at the diet. And when I gave in and ate the macaroni and cheese, I'd feel like a failure. Chances are I'd decide to eat the macaroni and cheese and stop following the diet. Knowing that I CAN eat macaroni and cheese makes it easier to CHOOSE NOT TO. I can say, "Not today. I'm going to treat myself next week," and not feel that I have been denied something because the power is mine. That said, I realize for some individuals certain foods are like what alcohol is to an alcoholic—one sip/bite and they will spiral out of control. If that applies to you, you may have to completely avoid that food. Similarly, some have health conditions that require limiting or eliminating specific foods. For the most part, though, you can find balance between being mastered by something and complete avoidance. So what does balance actually look like in practice?

For me, deal-breaker foods, ones I refuse to say I'm not allowed to or will never eat again, include french fries and sushi. So let's look at how I implement them in my diet.

Early on in my journey, I had the epiphany that, although white potatoes are not recommended for frequent consumption on the plan I follow, there is a big difference between having some and gluttony. In our culture, fries are served in gluttonous proportions in restaurants. From sit-down venues to fast-food joints, fries will comprise half or more of the meal in volume and nearly that much in calories. And we gobble them all down because to do otherwise would be a waste. Like consuming excess calories, which then get turned into fat on our bodies, isn't a waste? (Note sarcasm here.) Besides, they taste like heaven. It wouldn't take much to convince me they are laced with narcotics. But one day the light went on for me. How few fries could I eat and still feel satisfied? So, I started with ten. We do a family fry pile at fast-food places, so I'd count out 10 fries and set them with my meal. I could only eat those ten. Surprisingly, I found that I was okay with just 10, though it did take some time to break the habit of my hand just blindly reaching to the family pile during a meal because that's what you do when there are fries there. So, I wondered if I could get by with five. And voila, five was fine. That's where I settled. I order a meal with a side salad instead of fries, take my five fries from my kids' stash— I call it their "fry tax"—and am perfectly happy. Turns out, there is some science to back this up. The average calorie content of a medium order of fries at a fast-food restaurant is over 390 calories, and a large is over 500. And fries are the perfect mix of fat and high-glycemic carbohydrates that packs on pounds. However, the USDA recommended serving of fries is roughly the equivalent of 12-15 fries and has about 140 calories.[5] That's a big difference.

The other food I refuse to stop eating completely or find a healthy version of is sushi. White rice, and in particular the sticky white sushi rice, is not "allowed" in my new way of eating. It's high-glycemic and something that will send blood sugar swinging all over the place, which is one of the factors in fat storage. What's a sushi-loving girl to do? Thankfully, our budget limits our sushi consumption. That's a good start. We just can't afford to eat sushi, or at least good sushi, more often than every couple of months. There is also a Japanese dish called sashimi. It is the fish portion of sushi without the rice. Often it is served with grated daikon radish. Instead of a sushi platter, I now get a sushi/sashimi combo that has a few pieces of sushi roll, a couple pieces of sushi nigiri, and the remainder is sashimi. Balance.

Don't keep "forbidden" foods in your kitchen.
Do not buy foods to keep in the house or at your desk at work

that are not part of your plan, not even with the excuse that they are for your kids or your spouse. Treat those things like they are a fancy dish at a fancy restaurant, not something you'd make at home. This is how I approach macaroni and cheese now. I enjoy it from time to time (i.e. rarely) in a restaurant in moderation (i.e. I eat a few bites of it, not an entire bowl) and then go back to eating the way that is my new normal. I don't keep macaroni in my pantry at home because I have adopted the mindset of "I don't eat it," much like I don't buy peas to keep in my pantry because I don't eat them. I don't eat peas because they are disgusting, not because peas are not healthy, but you get the idea. We don't keep things we aren't going to eat in our homes so if we need to cut back on or eliminate a food from daily consumption not keeping it in the cupboard will go a long way in preventing a bad choice.

Know your plan's guidelines but don't be a slave to them.
Know how the choices you make will impact the results you want so you can make informed choices. Don't wait until you're sitting at Einstein Bros. for lunch with co-workers to try to figure out what you are going to eat there. Be familiar enough with the principles of the style of eating you have chosen so you can apply them anywhere. Just like you didn't memorize specific algebra problems in high school, you don't have to memorize every menu for every restaurant. In algebra, you learned *how* to solve the problem, so when the numbers changed, you could apply the method to solve the new problem. Same here. This is a big key to success. When real life hits, you have to be able to take the core principles and apply them to a less-than-ideal situation to come as close as possible to your plan. And, what is a good choice for you at one point in time may not be what the "right" choice is. There

may be nothing on a menu that is completely acceptable to your diet, and you just have to choose between the lesser of "evils." This is where grace and forgiveness come in. The next time you eat, you get to make another choice.

## Special occasions are not an excuse to "cheat."

Most of us have so many special occasions that if we "cheat" for every one of them, we'd spend very little time eating healthy. Between birthdays, anniversaries, holidays, dates with spouses, work celebrations, group meetings for Bible study or committees, etc. you can easily end up "cheating" several times a week rather than the more reasonable once a month. Figure out ahead of time what occasions you absolutely won't be able to stick to your plan for. My big one is Christmas, where I am visiting my parents, and my mom is doing the cooking. I don't expect her to cook to my diet, and I'm not going to insult her as a hostess by cooking my own things. So I'm prepared to make the best choices possible and have a few special holiday treats. Then I get back to my new habits at home. Then you have to set your mind that for all other special occasions you are going to have to follow your plan regardless of what others are doing.

## Don't beat yourself up when you do "cheat."

There will be times when you are forced to "cheat" by circumstances beyond your control. Or you may choose to "cheat" for whatever reason. Don't let those occasions convince you that you're a horrible person who is doomed to fail so you might as well give up. So you make one less than ideal decision; the next time you eat is another opportunity to make a better decision.

Finding your eating plan for life—the one that is right *for you*—is the key to this whole thing. Take the time to make your list of food issues. Make peace with the fact that there is no quick fix and that just because you saw your friend have great success on a certain plan doesn't mean it is the plan for you. Know that you're going to have to think about it and put some effort into learning new, better food habits. After a while, they will become just that, habits. It won't feel like work forever, but it does take some time. Look at it this way, a year from now you could be in the same place you are today. Or a year from now you can be that much closer to your goals. The choice is yours. You can do this.

# CHAPTER 4
# The Prison of Numbers

When my experiment had been underway for about two weeks, I went in for my yearly blood work and mammogram. I had said at the start that I would only weigh myself at the doctors' office, so while I was there, I popped in and asked if I could hop on the scale. I knew this was a dangerous idea. Weight doesn't go on overnight, and it doesn't come off overnight. Two weeks really wasn't that much time and, if there was no change, I was flirting with the temptation to give up. But I did it anyway. To my surprise, I had lost four pounds. Given that I was facing needing to lose more than 50 pounds, four pounds wasn't much, but at least I could see something was happening. Granted, I wasn't ready to give the diet credit just yet. I mean, four pounds in two weeks could easily be water weight, different clothing, different time of day, really just about anything. And therein lies a dieting dilemma— measuring success without becoming enslaved by numbers.

## The Scale
Of course, the first number that comes to mind when talking

about diet and body image is weight. So let's get real about that number. If the number on the scale is going down, we must be doing something right, and if it's going up, then we're failing yet again. Not so fast.

## The scale is just a number and has no real relation to your size or health It measures your gravitational pull to the earth and nothing else.

Weight is a complicated thing because it fluctuates so easily. If you weigh yourself every hour of the day, in your birthday suit, on the same scale, in the exact same location, you would find it goes up and down throughout the day. Typically, your weight will be the lowest first thing upon rising and increase over the course of the day. It will also vary over longer periods of time. For women, daily weights will fluctuate over the course of a month with their hormone cycle.

The dotted lines on the graphs below show my actual daily weights. The solid lines are the trend the app calculates based on patterns in the daily weights.[6] In the one month, graph you can see the dotted line is all over the map. Daily weights fluctuate based on cycle/hormone factors, water intake, exercise (strength training will cause you to retain a bit of water to help soothe those achy muscles), etc. Over three months though it evens out a little more. Over six months, it is even more smooth. And over one year, you see a trend like a straight decline; you can barely see the dotted line.

It is okay to weigh daily, but remember not to put too much stock in what that daily number is; it will change tomorrow. Actually, it will change ten seconds from now. What you ate yesterday may cause a short-term fluctuation in weight, but it is your LONG-TERM eating habits that are going to impact the trend of true weight gain or loss.

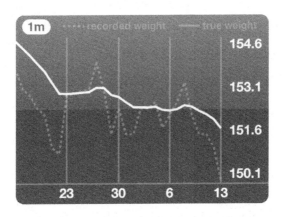

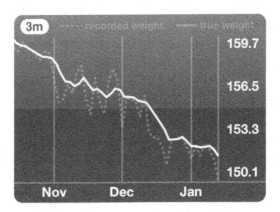

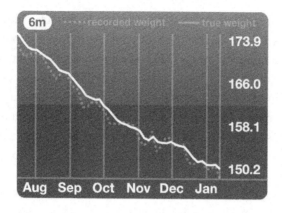

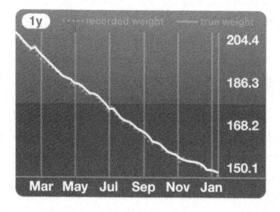

Weight also swings with the seasons. My eldest daughter works with horses. Every year in late July she tells me the horses look horrible because they are starting to bring in their winter coats. And every July this news makes me panic that the coming winter is going to be horrible. Why else would they be getting winter coats in July? But it turns out the seasonal coats of horses are driven by a very biological process related to the hours of daylight they are exposed to, not the temperature. When you stop to think about it, this makes sense. If the longest day of the year is in June, animals would need to start growing thicker fur when the days start getting noticeably shorter by the end of July. Only humans put on coats when it is already cold. Animals have to start the process when it's still warm because it takes time to grow a whole body of hair designed to protect against cold temperatures—particularly Minnesota-cold temperatures. Similarly, all vertebrates have what is called a hibernation cycle that is wired into their brains to slow metabolism and increase insulin-resistance to cause the body to store fat during winter months.[7]

How much the scale says you weigh has nothing to do with how you look. What weight looks like size-wise is influenced by things like how much of your body is muscle vs. fat and skeletal structure. You often hear people in dieting and health groups say things like, "A pound of muscle weighs less than a pound of fat." What they really mean is a pound of muscle takes up less physical space—is denser—than a pound of fat. One pound of muscle and one pound of fat weigh the same— a pound is a pound the world around—but muscle takes up drastically less space. People who have more muscle than fat are going to appear to weigh less because their muscles take up less room than an equivalent weight of fat.

Likewise, the same weight is going to look different, and register as a different clothing size, depending on body structure. It is entirely possible for six people to weigh exactly the same thing on the scale and actually look anywhere from slim and fit to frumpy and obese due to height, skeletal size, "apple" vs. "pear" shape, etc. And, as much as I hate to be the bearer of bad news, depending on what your body type and bone structure are, you may never have that flat stomach no matter how much weight you lose or how many sit-ups you do. Hey, don't shoot the messenger. I'm in the boat right along with y'all.

Weight is a perfectly valid measurement, but not for what we are using it to measure. Using weight to measure health and self-worth makes about as much sense as using a ruler to measure how hot it is outside. We need to start thinking of the number on the scale as how much the earth loves us rather than a commentary on our value, worth, or how healthy we are. That number, or a number based on it, does not tell the whole story about anyone.

## Body Mass Index

Because just measuring weight doesn't tell us much about health, doctors developed body mass index (BMI). BMI attempts to negate the problem of using weight alone to determine health by calculating a ratio of a person's weight in kilograms to their height in meters squared. For those of us who haven't gone metric yet, the equation gets even uglier.

$$\frac{mass_{lb}}{height_{in}^2} \times 703$$

That 703 is just the conversion ratio for getting from imperial/U.S. customary measurements to metric, but it still doesn't make it pretty.

There are several problems with BMI, starting with the fact that it is based on weight. As we've discussed, weight tells us nothing about muscle mass vs. fat mass, body frame size, etc. so basing another measurement on an already flawed measurement is not going to make a better measurement. And while BMI does attempt to take body frame size into consideration by factoring in height, it also fails to account for muscle mass or lack thereof.

We are told by mass media that a higher BMI puts us at risk for certain diseases, namely heart disease and diabetes. The reality is BMI itself does not put you at risk for or lessen your chances of anything. It's just a number. The reason BMI indicates risk factors for certain diseases is that the vast majority of overweight and obese people are eating the standard American, high-sugar, highly-processed diet. It is the sugar and processed food that puts them at risk for those diseases, not their weight or BMI. So, the high-sugar/highly-processed diet makes you fat (increases BMI because it increases your weight). And the high-sugar/highly-processed diet puts you at risk for diseases. The cause of the increased risk is not an increased BMI or weight. You can be "skinny fat." People who are skinny fat are those "lucky" ones who can eat the SAD/WPD diet of high-sugar and highly-processed food without putting on the pounds. They are thin and in the healthy BMI range but are still at risk for heart disease and diabetes. BMI may be a flashing red light to indicate a doctor should ask some questions about diet and other things to determine if there is a health risk, but BMI itself doesn't really indicate anything. Like weight, it's just a number.

## Clothing Sizes

After the scale, the next number we get all wrapped up in is our jean size or clothing size in general. As a side note, I'm old enough to remember that not too many years ago women defined themselves by dress size, now it's jean size. Hmm. The times they are a changin'.

Anyway, using clothing size alone to gauge weight loss success or justify your self-worth—for better or worse—is almost as bad as using weight. Women's clothing sizes vary widely from one brand to the next because they are non-standard. Sizes can measure significantly different even within the same brand and the same product. Part of the reason for this is the process used to cut the pieces for a garment. Stacks of fabric are punched out with dies. The natural compression and bending of the stack during the punching process can leave pieces on the top of the stack smaller than pieces on the bottom of the stack, sometimes by up to an inch.

I've heard many women wish that women's clothing was sized "standard" like men's. Your pant size would be measured by waist and inseam. Shirt size would be your neck or chest measurement. And it would be nice if it could work that way, but it can't. Owing to the wide variety of differences in women's shapes, it is possible for two women to have identical waists and inseams but not be able to wear the same size pants because of hips, or lack thereof, and other shape factors. That dratted body shape again. The other thing hindering this type of sizing for women would be the stigma women seem to have about telling people things like their waist size. Can you imagine how women would react to having anyone be able to find out their waist size just by being able to look at the tag in their jeans? I don't think it would go over well. Putting letters on clothes instead of numbers is no better. I own two belts. They are both a ladies' size XL. The smallest hole on the one is the same length from the buckle as the largest hole on the other. If I had been measuring success by what letter was stamped on the belt, I would have been pretty discouraged. And, in fact, I was at first—until I laid them side-by-side and saw how different they really were. Using clothing size as the sole method of measuring success in weight loss, we can be letting numbers and letters that are, quite literally, arbitrary run—or ruin—our lives.

## Mealtime Math Problems

There is one more way numbers can enslave us in the realm of eating. Many diets encourage or require some form of counting—calories, points, or macros (fats, carbohydrates, protein). This practice, in itself, isn't bad. However, because of the emotional high-stakes of weight loss and our human nature to believe that if we can control the numbers we can control the outcome, what starts off as a way to help us make good choices can quickly become a prison of mealtime number-crunching that slowly drives us, and those around us, crazy. It is wise to be cognizant of abusing calories and to monitor macro ratios, but we must be careful that in doing so we don't become enslaved to it. I personally don't count anything. Not even fries really. When I say five fries, it isn't always exactly five. Five fries is a principle for me, not a number. I guess I technically count the hours between eating times. I make sure I'm leaving three to four hours, allowing my body time to use what I've given it. That is all I count. As I mentioned in the previous chapter, I favor keeping a simple food diary, with two exceptions.

The first exception is when you are just getting started. It can be helpful to do some counting in those early weeks to get an idea of just how many calories various foods have or what foods are carbs vs. fats vs. proteins. But once you have a basic idea of those things, counting should fall by the wayside. I would say counting should not last more than six to eight weeks but that time frame will, of course, vary by person. By counting, I'm not meaning doing a detailed recording with an app or complicated measuring, weighing, and calculating at every meal. I'm saying have a look at the nutrition label on a package, note the serving size, and get an idea of how many calories, carbs, fats, and protein are in that serving size. Then do a mental measurement of how much you ate. Your clenched fist is roughly equal to 1 cup. A cupped palm is about 1/2 cup. Your thumb approximately 1 tablespoon. And, the tip of the thumb to the first joint is about 1 teaspoon.

The second scenario when counting might be called for is if you find, or suspect you have, a serious problem with calorie abuse. By serious problem, I mean bordering on eating disorder level calorie abuse. *Occasionally* eating seconds or eating more than a serving size of ice cream is normal. Having seconds or thirds (or more) at every meal is calorie abuse. Eating a pint or more every time you have ice cream is calorie abuse. Even eating healthy foods in excess signals an unhealthy relationship with food. And, eating excess amounts of healthy foods can cause weight gain or inhibit weight loss. Just because it's healthy doesn't mean it doesn't impact the calories in/calories out balance. If this is you, counting and measuring portions may be something you need to do, for a time. However, I would also encourage you to seek professional help to deal with whatever is fueling your tendency to abuse calories. And don't remain in the counting and measuring camp forever. When you see success come after counting and measuring, it can be easy and tempting to turn counting and measuring into a god of sorts. Thinking that controlling the numbers is the be-all, end-all to success is a trap. It quickly becomes a prison that controls you. What do you do when you eat at a restaurant where calorie counts aren't available? You spend your whole meal inputting the info into an app to calculate it rather than enjoying the company of those you are eating with. That's not controlling the numbers; that's the numbers controlling you. It's not worth it to constantly be worrying about the numbers.

## Getting Real and Staying Out of Number Prison

Staying out of number prison is a lot like finding the best diet. It is critical to know yourself—your emotional attachment to the scale number, how you feel about your clothing size, how fast you think weight should come off, and just how much you believe controlling life's numbers will guarantee a specific outcome.

### Set realistic weight and clothing size goals.

What you want to see on the scale as your ideal weight may not actually be your ideal weight but an unrealistic idea of what you think is right. What jean size you want to be may not be the jean size you are supposed to be. My personal belief is whatever you are happy with when you look in the mirror is what your ideal weight or clothing size is, regardless of what number appears on the scale or is printed on the tag of your clothing. Of course, that makes it hard to measure because you don't know what that number or size is until you get there.

### Stay off the scale for AT LEAST six weeks when starting a new way of eating.

Losing weight takes time. As you can see in the graphs above, the short-term fluctuations can give the appearance that nothing is happening. This causes a lot of people to give up before things really get started. Give yourself time to learn new habits, give your body time to adjust to those new habits, and stay off the scale for six weeks. Take a starting weight and then hide your scale if that's what it takes to stay off it.

### Take measurements in addition to weighing.

At a minimum, take chest/bust, waist, and hip measurements. This helps you keep track of progress that may not show on the scale. If you are strength training, for example, you may not see much in the way of scale progress, but measuring will show that you are slimming down because of the loss of fat and gaining of muscle.

### Expect and don't be in a hurry to break scale "stalls."

Chances are, at some point in your journey, you will experience a "stall." This is a period of time when the scale sits at roughly the same number—you're no longer seeing a downward trend—for weeks or months, and it's not your goal weight. They seem to happen about every 20 pounds or so for a lot of people in weight loss mode, though it varies from person to person. Many experience their first stall, conclude they have failed, and simply give up. They go back to their destructive habits, gaining back what they have lost and often packing on some additional as well. Others frantically search for a way to "break" the stall. They start severely restricting calories, switch diets, and/or exercise more, all in an attempt to get the scale showing a downward trend again. Stalls can be particularly discouraging unless you know they are coming and that your body needs them. Plan for them. Don't rush to break them. When you have stalls, your body is doing other things—resting, healing, tightening up skin. Let it. Stick to your new habits and see what happens.

Set small goals as you go rather than a big end goal.

Don't start out with an ending number or size set in stone. When I started, I didn't set a weight goal at all. I had no idea what a reasonable weight was for me. After almost 20 years and three babies, it seemed unrealistic to expect to get back to what I weighed in college. Charts can give some idea of what your weight should be given gender, height, and skeletal frame size, but they aren't always the most accurate. So, if you have to set a goal weight, start with a small step. Depending on where you start, this will be 5 or 10 pounds. I wouldn't go higher than a loss of 10 pounds as your first goal for weight. When you meet that goal, evaluate how you're feeling physically, how you're feeling emotionally about what you see in the mirror, what size clothing you're wearing, and then set another small goal.

Keep the majority of your goals non-scale goals.

All of the initial goals I wrote down were non-scale ones—things like lower blood lipid numbers, lower blood pressure, being able to wear my wedding ring again, smaller clothing sizes. I have heard people set goals like being able to fly without needing a seatbelt extender, being able to ride a roller coaster, fitting into stadium seats at sporting events, or shopping in stores that don't carry plus sizes. As your journey progresses, keep an eye out for non-scale victories. Many of them will be things that never crossed your mind until you suddenly realize they are different. I vividly remember the day I noticed my thighs no longer rubbed together when I walked, the evening I walked up two flights of stairs in a parking garage without being winded, and seeing the seat of the car between my knees when driving. It's the little things, folks. You'll amass quite a collection of these non-scale milestones, but if you're too focused on the scale number, you'll miss them and the joy they provide.

*Know how the scale number impacts you mentally and emotionally and use the scale accordingly.*

My original intent was to only weigh at my doctor's office. At some point, I did start weighing weekly at home. Then, for two weeks in a row, my husband and I weighed exactly the same thing. That seemed really odd, and we suspected our scale was not functioning properly. Being geeks, we realized the only way to know would be for each of us to weigh every day and note if the trend continued. So we changed the batteries in the scale and grabbed a pad of paper. After a couple weeks, we did get a new scale, but daily weighing had become a habit. It was interesting from a data standpoint, so I kept doing it.

There are multiple schools of thought on how often you should weigh. Daily weighing gives you a lot of data; it will show trends over time. You can use knowledge of trends to help you evaluate progress. On the other hand, weight swings, sometimes wildly, from one day to the next. Seeing an increase from the previous day can freak some people out. Here's the deal, if what number you see every morning is going to make or break your day, you need to decide how to deal with it, or it will turn your journey into a rollercoaster ride from hell. You can opt not to weigh every day. Some people don't weigh at all. Or you can weigh daily but use it as a way to overcome your reactions to the fluctuations, kind of a DIY a form of exposure therapy or cognitive behavioral therapy.

There are many days, even and maybe especially now at goal weight, where I see the scale number and cringe. There are mornings it's up, sometimes over a pound. I have to remind myself to take a deep breath, calm down, and think rationally. Then I walk through the following thought process. First, God is where I get my value, not the scale. I pray for peace and calm. In the grand scheme of things, and even in the tiny little corner of the universe that is my life, what I see on the scale is NOT what matters. Second, that number will be different tomorrow. And in all likelihood, tomorrow's number will be lower. Then, what has my trend been? Have I seen increases for several days in a row? What season is it? Humans naturally put on weight during the winter. Next, what has my diet been like lately? Have I been sticking to my new eating habits or have I been moderating myself out of moderation? Did I have a particularly salty meal? Did I attend a special event and treat myself to something that would cause water retention? Fifth, did I do anything physically stressful beyond my normal workout? As I write this, we are having a record year for snow here in the Midwest and Great Plains. I'm blessed to have a husband and a snowblower to deal with snowpocalypse. However, while dog-sitting one weekend, I had to shovel a couple inches of snow, twice. Shoveling uses different muscle groups in different ways than I'm used to. That leads to a degree of water retention by the body to soothe those muscles that aren't used to working so hard. The result, the scale was up for a day or two. How are my clothes fitting—tighter than normal or the same as usual? Awkward but other valid considerations: How are my bowel habits? Where am I in my hormone cycle? Up a couple pounds or more just prior to menstruation is normal. Finally, am I making excuses or deluding myself in any way? As always, honest answers are necessary. By the time I've walked through prayer and logical considerations, I'm off the edge of the "I'M-GOING-TO-GAIN-IT-ALL-BACK-AND-BE-FAT-AGAIN-SO-I-THINK-I'LL-CURL-UP-IN-A-FETAL-POSITION-AND-CRY-ALL-DAY!!!" cliff. I can rest in the peace of knowing God is my strength and my weight just a number, as well as having insight into anything I might need to address. All that said, this process doesn't work for some people unless they have help in it, so they will either need to avoid the scale or get help in dealing with it. There is nothing to be ashamed of if that is the case. We all have things we just can't overcome or deal with on our own. Admitting you need and seeking help for those things is not a sign of weakness or failure but actually shows a great deal of strength.

Numbers in weight loss can be helpful tools for evaluating progress on the journey. However, it is important to keep them in perspective to avoid ending up being enslaved by them. Numbers give us an illusion of control. We believe that if we can control the numbers, we can control our lives. They make us feel safe. But tying our achievements and self-worth to those numbers makes us slaves to them.

# CHAPTER 5
# Move It!

Three months into my journey, I got the following text from my sister:

1/30/16, 5:47 PM

> Hey! I know you said you're not wanting to work out but let me know if you would want to maybe walk a 5k "race". Mary and I are trying to do one race every month this year. I think it would be fun to do together! Maybe we could get together and walk on the weekends? If you're totally not interested though that's OK...just tell me to get lost!

Here's the deal with my sister and exercise: she is a runner—like she's done half marathons. And she does all those exercise things like boot camp and kettlebell workouts. And she does them really early in the morning. I'm pretty sure she has memberships at multiple gyms. Here's the deal with me and exercise: I don't. The Trim Healthy Mama authors recommend not starting a new exercise program while simultaneously undertaking THM as a new way of eating. I took them seriously. Actually, I had taken this recommendation and read it as "don't exercise if you don't want to," which is not what it said. I know exercise is physically good for me. I know it will improve my mental and emotional wellbeing. But a stellar lack of physical coordination, a love of lounging, and vivid memories of being made fun of in physical education in junior high made it sink to near the bottom of my priority list. A root canal might have ranked higher. So when a book on weight loss tells you not to start an exercise program when you start their eating plan, it sounds like music to your lazy ears. However, by the time I received my sister's text, I had lost about 20 pounds. I'd been feeling like I should be doing some kind of exercise. So, in a moment of weakness, I answered her with:

1/30/16, 8:22 PM

I was thinking about that the other day. If I start now, I might be ready to do one come September/October. Maybe for my 43rd birthday!

I told my husband, "I think I just agreed to do a 5k with my sister."

His reply, "You can't do that! It will kill you!"

Gee thanks, dear. Of course, that meant I had to do it.

My daughter told me, in that know-it-all way teens have, "You're going to end up doing them for fun."

"No, I'm not," I argued and waved an emphatic index finger at her, "I agreed to one. One!"

I've seen various numbers tossed around by experts on weight loss about how much of losing weight is the result of diet vs. exercise. Some claim it's 80% nutrition and 20% exercise. Some say 70/30, others 75/25. There doesn't seem to be a hard set of numbers to settle on. But one thing is clear, weight loss depends largely on changing eating habits and reducing calorie intake and is less impacted by working out. There are two reasons for this. First, exercise doesn't burn as many calories as you think it does. For instance, walking one mile results in burning about 100 calories—give or take. Considering there are 3,500 calories in one pound of fat, 100 calories seems like hardly a dent. Second, you need to use the calories you consume within a time frame of about three to four hours, or the extra calories will be stored as fat. Stored fat likes to stay put. One Starbucks Tall (12 ounce) Caffe Latte made with 2% milk has 150 calories.[8] So for every Caffe Latte, you drink you need to walk 1.5 miles to burn off its calories. And, you need to take that walk within four hours, not at the end of the day or the next morning. It's easier to not drink the Caffe Latte than it is to walk the extra mile within a few hours of drinking it.

That doesn't mean you shouldn't exercise. Even those of us who are, ahem, "allergic" to exercise need to exercise, at least a little bit. Since I'm not big into exercise, I don't have a whole lot of advice for you on this subject. What little I do have probably falls into the category of "well, duh," but here it goes.

**Don't start a new exercise routine at the same time you start a new way of eating.**

There are two reasons for this. First, it is hard enough to learn new eating habits. If you try to incorporate new exercise habits at the same time, your chances of getting frustrated with both and throwing in the towel on both increases. Additionally, when starting out with new exercise regimens, your body will go through a rebellion of sorts. The exercise will cause a small amount of inflammation initially. This will result in the retention of water and, therefore, a temporary increase in weight. Also, an increase in physical activity will actually signal your body to hang on to weight for a little while. It has to decide if you're serious about this and realize it isn't going to starve before it gets on board with letting go of extra weight. A similar thing happens when you start new eating habits. Your body has a bit of a panic attack before it gets on board with the new way of eating. It hangs on to weight until it realizes you aren't depriving it of things it needs. So if you start the two things at the same time, it will take longer to see results. And if you start strength training, it will build muscle, which will give an appearance of no weight loss on the scale. In actuality, the muscle you build in strength training takes up less space than the same weight of fat, so you are getting smaller even though the scale doesn't show it.

Find the right exercise for you.
Like diets, there is no one best exercise. What the right exercise is for you depends on many things specific to you.

∂　Know your goals. Weight loss isn't really a realistic goal for exercise. It will help weight loss but, as noted above, exercise itself isn't going to result in significant weight reduction. There are other aspects of health exercise can have a big impact on though. And if you want to target a specific goal, you'll want to select a type of exercise suited to that goal. Here are a few of the goals that exercise will help:

- Increased strength/muscle
- Heart conditioning
- Endurance
- Lowering LDL and/or increasing HDL
- Improving moods/emotions and mental wellness

∂   Know what you like to do. Knowing what you enjoy and how your body reacts to different kinds of activity can help you pick the right thing for you. Personally, I can't stand to have my arms extended away from my body for more than a couple inches (yes, I have issues). This means that things like weights, Zumba, kettlebell, and most group exercise classes aren't something I'm going to enjoy, not to mention the fact that, as I noted previously, the instructor's life would be in danger from me the second time she said, "Keep going! Just five more!" in that gym instructor voice. Likewise, my ability to follow mentally and physically at the same time makes team sports not a good idea. Walking and running are good things for me. They don't require any particular skills or coordination or much thought. Although I did manage to do a face plant on the sidewalk one morning while doing my cool-down walk after a run, so I might not even really have enough coordination for them. But I digress... Exercise doesn't have to be *exercise*—as in going to the gym, lifting weights, Zumba classes, running, etc. It just has to be something that gets you moving. A few ideas:

- Biking
- Horseback riding

- Swimming
- Gardening
- Yoga

∂ Know your habits or lack thereof. The best exercise for you is what you are going to do regularly. Maybe for you that isn't necessarily one thing. I'm a creature of habit and routine, bordering a bit on autistic that way. I have eaten cinnamon granola for breakfast every day for over a year. I do my grocery shopping every Thursday morning. I do the same workout on the same mornings each week. But that's just me. Some people are all about variety and are very spontaneous about life. If that's you, maybe you want to swim some days and work in the garden on others. The big thing is that you get 150 minutes of moderate physical activity per week. How you divide that up is up to you, though it is suggested to get at least 30 minutes per day most days of the week.[9]

∂ Know your health limitations. Some health limitations are temporary. When I started exercising, I was still pretty heavy—over 200 pounds. My knees and ankles ached a lot with very little physical activity. As more weight came off and I built up muscles that hadn't been used regularly for a long time, walking and jogging hurt less and less. So, what your limitations are at one point may not be what they are later. You may want to start with something low-impact like swimming and then move to higher impact things as you lose more weight. However, other health issues like heart conditions or arthritis may impose long-term or permanent limitations. It is likely though there is some kind of physical activity you can do despite your limitations. No, it might not be running a marathon or even walking a 5k, but there is something that you can do no matter how small. And, something is better than nothing. IMPORTANT: If you haven't seen a doctor in a while (and even if you have) it is a good idea to do so before undertaking new exercises.

So, what became of that 5k with my sister? Well, it didn't kill me as my husband predicted it would. As much as it pains me to admit that my teenager was right, it did turn into me doing them for fun. My sister patiently walked the first one with me about four months after our texts. My youngest got on board with the running. She was lured in by the "free" t-shirts, though in her case they actually are free because I pay her race registration fees. We started jogging two mornings a week. Then we ran (I use the term loosely, I'm a slow runner) part of a 5k three months later. And then there was a Turkey Trot. The next year we did five more. And the year after that another four. This year, I ran a 6.5-mile leg of a marathon relay as part of a four-person team. I'll probably do at least three 5ks with my daughter as well. Never in a million years did I think I'd actually *want* to do any physical activity. Now I find myself saying things like, "I really need to go for a run," and not in the same way I'd say, "I really need to dust behind the fridge," but meaning that my body is physically hungering for it. You just never know what you'll end up enjoying.

# CHAPTER 6
# With Friends Like That...

Fourteen months into my journey, Christmas had rolled around again. This meant a trip to see both my extended family as well as my in-laws. I hadn't told anyone besides my husband, kids, and Bible study group that I was eating differently or trying to lose weight. I just couldn't face all the knowing looks that silently said, "Good luck with that," or mounds of unsolicited advice on how to accomplish it. For me, this was an experiment to see if the THM method really worked. And if it didn't, I didn't want to be hearing all the out loud or implied criticism. We've all had that friend, or maybe have even been that person, who enthusiastically declares, to the point of being somewhat annoying, that they are going to get in shape and drop the weight and, six months later, nothing has happened. I didn't want to be that person. I couldn't deal with getting my hopes up only to have them dashed, and I certainly couldn't deal with disapproval or judgment from others.

The visit began with Christmas Eve at my in-laws'. My husband's family is Scandinavian and from a small town in

South Dakota. In case you are unfamiliar with how small-town Scandinavian South Dakotans work, they talk a lot about the weather, what they had for dinner last night, the latest community happenings, and how the local high school sports teams are doing. Surface talk. So, there I got, "You look great," but that's it. I wasn't expecting and didn't want much else. My family is less Scandinavian but just as small-town South Dakotan. I wasn't even expecting a "You look great," there. Not that they wouldn't think it, they just don't say things like that. But when we arrived at my parents' and I walked into their kitchen, my aunt was speechless. Well, nearly speechless. I believe she said something along the lines of, "Wow!" Once she had recovered a bit, she added, "How much weight have you lost?!?" I didn't lose the weight to get reactions or attention or prove anything to anyone but myself. But I have to admit, that reaction did make me feel more pleased than I should have let it for a couple reasons. First, my aunt is not often speechless. I knew I looked quite a bit different, but since I see myself every day, I didn't really think about how people who don't see me very often would notice the change all at once. I hadn't seen my aunt since the previous Christmas, so it was quite a shock for her. And then there was just a bit of pride. I had lost almost 70 pounds and, dang it, it was nice to have someone make kind of a big deal about it. However, in one of those strange paradoxes of life, people making a big deal about it would quickly become kind of old too.

## How Did You Lose So Much Weight?

One of the first things others seem to want to know is what you are doing to have noticeable success at weight loss. When they ask, we get all excited and start giving them a monologue on all the ins and outs of our particular diet plan. When you find something that works and changes your life so dramatically, you want to share it with everyone. However, most people don't want to hear what you really did. They are hoping you found some magic that made it easy. It has been my experience when people ask how I've done it, and I tell them "I separate fats from carbs," and "I no longer eat sugar," I see their expressions change as they realize it involved significant changes in eating habits. What they are looking for is a quick fix (if weight is an issue for them). When I can't offer that it's almost as if they think I'm talking about rocket science that they can't possibly hope to accomplish. I'm now at the point that, when people ask how I've lost so much weight, I just say I follow an eating plan called Trim Healthy Mama and leave it at that. If they want to know more, I let them ask. If their eyes glaze over, I drop the subject. I've planted the seed. The seed will grow if/when it is the right time for that person.

## Here, Have a Cookie. One Won't Kill You

I refer to this as others trying to force-feed you. I have only encountered this occasionally, but other people I know have had to endure it far more often. Also, it seems to be a particular problem for women who are losing weight and is perpetrated by women toward those who are losing. Men don't seem to do this, or at least they don't do it as much as women do. It is often a problem at gatherings like family holiday celebrations or office parties. You know how it goes. Your mother (or sister or co-worker or great-aunt or sister-in-law or next-door neighbor or…) offers you her world-famous triple-chocolate fudge cake with a scoop of ice cream. You respond with a polite, "No, thank you." She may know you are working on changing your eating habits, she may not, but she is not going to take, "No, thank you," for an answer. Often, if she does know you are trying to eat better, she'll break out the phrases, "One isn't going to kill you," or "It's okay to enjoy yourself once in a while." For some reason, people seem to think if you are eating healthier, you must also be miserable. However, if you have selected an eating plan that is suited to your preferences for food, you should not be miserable eating healthy. Additionally, while it's true that one isn't going to kill you, depending on your food issues, one might set off a spiral that lasts far longer than just one—in effect meaning that one may indeed kill your success. If people said the same type of thing to an alcoholic—"Just one sip or one beer isn't going to kill you."—others would be appalled. (Though, sadly, I'm sure there are people who say such things to alcoholics.)

So, you have two choices. One, you can do the Minnesota-nice thing we do where I live and cave in and accept it. This will get her to leave you alone and avoid hurting her feelings. Or you can stay strong, and maybe even become a bit "firm" in your refusal. This may result in you being labeled as a rude [word that rhymes with witch]. Personally, I'm a fan of adopting the attitude of, "Other people are not in charge of what *I* eat." I use a mix of firm niceness and decline with a polite, "No, thank you," as many times as it takes. It seems that the unwritten rule is they'll ask three times and then give up. If their feelings get hurt because I don't eat the cake they made, too bad. That's their problem. However, other people may have deep-seated relationship issues with people that exhibit this behavior toward them on their journey. And others may have such an uncontrollable desire to please others that they can't continue to refuse for fear of upsetting the offerer.

If you are in a situations like those, you may need to seek help working through the relationship dynamic or your people pleasing nature. That will allow you to healthily say, "I'm in charge of what I eat, not you," and not be victim to emotional or psychological abuse from that person's reaction to you standing up for yourself. And there are situations where sometimes you have to take a deep breath and eat the cake (or whatever it is). If you only see your mother-in-law twice a year, her feelings may be crushed if you don't eat a meal she prepared specifically for your visit. So, you sit down, eat whatever she made in moderation, say a prayer of thanksgiving that you have a meal to eat and can spend time with family, and rest in the assurance that the next time you eat is an opportunity to make good choices. That one meal with your mother-in-law won't kill you, or at least not for nutrition reasons. But if you eat at your mother-in-law's every Sunday then you have to set boundaries.

As I mentioned, this does seem to largely be a behavior that is a woman thing. Maybe it's the result of centuries of women being the ones primarily responsible for cooking and feeding those around us. It's how we are taught to be hospitable to guests. It could just be that, as a woman, I hear stories about it from women more than men. I do suspect though there is some degree of gender difference in how men and women react to losing weight and to the weight loss of others. I'm not alone. A male friend who has also lost a significant amount of weight, and incidentally has a master's degree in Christian counseling, shared how he has experienced the reactions of others to his weight loss. Interestingly enough, he felt that women tended to be more supportive of each other when someone they knew was losing weight and that men felt a degree of conviction and/or shame when they saw a friend make healthy choices and drop weight because they know they should be doing likewise. Being on the woman side of the coin, I suspect women feel conviction and/or shame when seeing the success of another like men do but become passive-aggressive and self-shaming in their reaction to those emotions. If you're a woman, you know how this works. Mary runs into Suzie at the PTA meeting. "Hey, Suzie! You're looking so fabulous! How much have you lost?!? Good for you!" And then five minutes later, out of earshot of Suzie, "Ashley, did you see Suzie? How long do you suppose it'll be before she gains it all back? Honestly, I liked her better fat. …" Or instead of gossiping, Mary goes home and cries all night because she feels like a big fat failure compared to Suzie. And in reality, Mary probably both gossips and cries all night. Men, on the other hand, tend to deal with their reaction by not dealing with it.

## Can We Please Talk About Something Else?

One reaction I get far more often is that my weight loss and its side effects (my doing 5ks and such) are ALL we end up talking about. And while it is flattering and can be fun to talk about, it does get old after a while. As thrilled as I am with it, it's not the only thing in my life. I want to share something like, "I did a 5k and finished in my best time ever," have them say, "Congrats," and move on. It gets old when people comment about it every time they see you.

Weight loss is a very emotional thing. When it is going well, your emotions soar; you feel good about yourself and what you've accomplished. When it is a struggle, your emotions tank, and you feel as if you are a complete failure. These are very natural and automatic human reactions to success or failure at anything. And just like success or failure at other things, the reactions of those around us can compound the intensity of these emotions. It is important to remember that you can only control *your* reactions; you can't control the reactions of others. Equally significant is that their reactions have nothing to do with you. The reactions of others are rooted in things going on in their lives or struggles they are having (and not necessarily weight loss ones) that likely don't have anything to do with you.

# CHAPTER 7
# Joy In The Journey

Two years after beginning, I officially closed my experiment. The end of the experiment wasn't the end of my diet, just the end of taking monthly pictures and record keeping. My new way of eating is now truly a habit. The way I think about food and how I eat is different and automatic. I will honestly say that when I stopped the experiment part, I believed I was at my body's goal weight. The scale had been showing the same number for weeks. Others have asked why I felt it was where my body was settling and not a weight-loss stall. The answer is simple. It was where my body was comfortable, as well as my mind. I had lost 80 pounds and was perfectly happy with how I felt and looked. My medical numbers were good, and I had always felt that when my body stopped losing, where it stopped would be my goal weight. Secretly though, I had an unspoken goal weight I kind of wanted to reach. But it was only five pounds lower, so I was okay not reaching it. However, seven months later, with no additional changes to my routine or intentional attempt to lose more, I reached my unspoken goal weight for a total loss of 85 pounds. I could probably go militant and lose enough to get as low as I was in high school or college, but it would be at the cost of my joy and freedom. Since I now wear a size smaller than I did in either high school or college even though I weigh 10 pounds more, I don't feel the need to go down that road. I opt for freedom and joy.

Now that I have been in maintenance mode for a little over a year, I will say that maintenance mode is a bit more stressful for me than loss mode. Maintenance mode typically involves a range of about ten pounds weight swings around in; it isn't just one number. Mine is no exception. My target is 135, and some days I'm up around 138; other days, I can be in the 132 neighborhood.

Still, there is an ever-present nagging in my mind that I could gain it all back. And, honestly, it terrifies me. I was miserable, and I have no desire to be miserable again. As I mentioned before, being thin will not make you happy, and it hasn't made me happy. Don't get me wrong, I like being thinner. But it's the healthy changes I have made, coupled with the mental and emotional issues I've worked through as part of that change process, that have improved my quality of life. If I had gotten my original wish of just miraculously waking up 100 pounds lighter one morning, I would have missed the real benefits that weight loss held for me, which were really not about weight at all.

There you have it. All the secrets I can give you about weight loss. While they can't guarantee success, I do believe that they can help you on your journey. Remember, there is no best diet, quick fix, magic formula, or guarantees. Anyone who tries to tell you otherwise is trying to sell you something. Stay honest with yourself. Look at your personal preferences, motivations, and history to guide you in what the best diet, best exercise, and realistic goals are for you. Stay hopeful. You are not alone in the journey. Find a support system. It may be one person; it may be a group. It may be in person; it may be on-line. It may change from season to season as you move along your journey. The kind of support you need at the start may give way to needing a different kind as you progress. But, sharing your story with and hearing the stories of others who are on the same journey helps us all on our way. In particular, it helps to find a group that is following the same eating style you have chosen. The Trim Healthy Mama Facebook group provided me with invaluable support and resources, especially during the first 18 months or so. Stay sane. Weight loss is a formidable opponent, particularly when you are starting out. It can be very easy to get sucked into a place where your diet and exercise take over your entire life. I know. I've been there. When you're eating, you're focused on making the right choices. When you're not eating, you're thinking about when and what you'll be eating next, and how it fits in your plan. When you're not thinking about when and what to eat, you're learning and talking about your eating plan so you know how to make good choices. This is all very common and somewhat necessary when you're new on the journey. The problem is, after a while, this immersion can become a habit, and before you know it, you find every waking moment is being consumed by a good thing that has now become an obsession. It is important to learn to walk the line between being mindful and being obsessed. After about 18 months, I realized that I was heading toward obsession, spending way too much time with my Facebook support group discussing the ins and outs of THM. As much as I appreciated the insight and support I found there, it was overtaking my life. I liked being able to give back by helping others that were new to it. But, spending every free minute I had answering questions at the group, and getting caught up in debates over minute details, was draining and causing me to neglect other things I enjoyed. It is important to have a support system, but it is equally important not to rely on them to the exclusion of having a life. Being zeroed in on a goal is great, but if it is all you think about and work toward, things are out of balance. Life will pass you by while you're thinking, "When I get to xxx pounds, I'll take the kids to the pool and actually get in it with them," or "When I can buy x size jeans, I'll be happy." Do those things now! Be happy in the process. You only get one chance. You may get to your goals quickly. You may never get there. "The race is long and, in the end, it's only with yourself."[10] Have some good memories to hang on to when you get there!

Don't let food rule your life! Choose joy!

# End Notes

CHAPTER 2

[1] Ducharme, Jamie. "About Half of Americans Say They're Trying to Lose Weight." *Time*, 12 July 2018, time.com/5334532/weight-loss-americans/.

Searing, Linda. "The Big Number: 45 Million Americans Go on a Diet Each Year." *The Washington Post*, WP Company, 1 Jan. 2018, www.washingtonpost.com/national/health-science/the-big-number-45-million-americans-go-on-a-diet-each-year/2017/12/29/04089aec-ebdd-11e7-b698-91d4e35920a3_story.html?utm_term=.ddbe52538f41.

Freedhof, Yoni. "No, 95 Percent of People Don't Fail Their Diets." *U.S. News & World Report*, U.S. News & World Report, 17 Nov. 2014, health.usnews.com/health-news/blogs/eat-run/2014/11/17/no-95-percent-of-people-dont-fail-their-diets.

Fildes, Alison, et al. "Probability of an Obese Person Attaining Normal Body Weight: Cohort Study Using Electronic Health Records." *American Journal of Public Health*, vol. 105, no. 9, Sept. 2015, doi:10.2105/ajph.2015.302773.

Wolpert, Stuart. "Dieting Does Not Work, UCLA Researchers Report." *UCLA Newsroom*, UCLA, 3 Apr. 2007, newsroom.ucla.edu/releases/Dieting-Does-Not-Work-UCLA-Researchers-7832.

[2] Tapp, Teresa. *What's Your Body Type?*, www.t-Tapp.com.

## CHAPTER 3

[3] LaRosa, John. "Top 6 Trends for the Weight Loss Industry in 2018." *Market Research Blog*, MarketResearch.com, 2 Jan. 2018, blog.marketresearch.com/top-6-trends-for-the-weight-loss-market-in-2018.

[4] *JAMA Intern Med.* Published online September 12, 2016. doi:10.1001/jamainternmed.2016.5394. *JAMA Intern Med.* 2016;176(11):1680-1685. doi:10.1001/jamainternmed.2016.5394.

[5] Average medium french fry calories determined using data from:

> *Burger King USA Nutritionals*, Burger King Corporation, Apr. 2019, www.bk.com/pdfs/nutrition.pdf.

> "Chick-Fil-A Waffle-Potato-Fries." *Chick-Fil-A.com*, Chick-Fil-A, Inc., 2019, www.chick-fil-a.com/Menu-Items/Waffle-Potato-Fries.

> "Culver's Nutrition Grid & Facts." *Culvers.com*, Culver Franchising System, LLC, 2019, www.culvers.com/menu-and-nutrition/nutrition-grid.

> "Hardee's Nutrition Information." *Hardees.com*, Hardee's Restaurants, LLC, 2019, www.hardees.com/nutrition.

> "McDonald's Nutrition Calculator." *McDonald's*, McDonald's Corporation, 2019, www.mcdonalds.com/us/en-us/about-our-food/nutrition-calculator.html.

> "Natural Cut Fries – Wendy's." *Wendys.com*, Quality Is Our Recipe, LLC, 2017,

menu.wendys.com/en_US/product/french-fries/.

Mele, Christopher. "You Don't Want Fries With That." *The New York Times*, The New York Times, 29 Nov. 2018, www.nytimes.com/2018/11/29/health/french-fries-nutrition.html.

Nicola Veronese, Brendon Stubbs, Marianna Noale, Marco Solmi, Alberto Vaona, Jacopo Demurtas, Davide Nicetto, Gaetano Crepaldi, Patricia Schofield, Ai Koyanagi, Stefania Maggi, Luigi Fontana; Fried potato consumption is associated with elevated mortality: an 8-y longitudinal cohort study, *The American Journal of Clinical Nutrition*, Volume 106, Issue 1, 1 July 2017, Pages 162–167, https://doi.org/10.3945/ajcn.117.154872.

## CHAPTER 4

[6] O'Bryan, Rory. "True Weight." *True Weight*, 2016, www.madeupsoftware.com/trueweight/home.html.

[7] Hatipoglu, Betul. "Hibernation Mode Slows Metabolism During Fall and Winter Seasons." *U.S. News & World Report*, U.S. News & World Report, 10 Dec. 2015, health.usnews.com/health-news/patient-advice/articles/2015/12/10/hibernation-mode-slows-metabolism-during-fall-and-winter-seasons.

Chronic Conditions Team. "How the Seasons Can Affect Your Body's Metabolism." *Health Essentials from Cleveland Clinic*, Health Essentials from Cleveland Clinic, 17 Dec. 2015, health.clevelandclinic.org/how-the-seasons-can-affect-your-bodys-metabolism/.

## CHAPTER 5

[8] "Explore Our Menu." *Starbucks Coffee Company*, Starbucks Coffee Company, 2019, www.starbucks.com/menu/catalog/nutrition?drink=all#view_control=nutrition.

[9] Laskowski, Edward R. "How Much Exercise Do You Really Need?" *Mayo Clinic*, Mayo Foundation for Medical Education and Research, 27 Apr. 2019, www.mayoclinic.org/healthy-lifestyle/fitness/expert-answers/exercise/faq-20057916.

## CHAPTER 7

[10] Schmich, Mary. "Advice, like Youth, Probably Just Wasted on the Young." *Chicagotribune.com*, Chicago Tribune, 1 June 1997, www.chicagotribune.com/news/columnists/chi-schmich-sunscreen-column-column.html.

# Acknowledgements

My husband, Keith, has been my biggest supporter and encourager in all my adult endeavors. I could not have asked for a better life partner.

Abigail, Emily, and Ingrid make motherhood look easy. I'm blessed beyond measure to be trusted with the job of guiding them into becoming respectable human beings.

Well, you see, my sister... Sandy Kruse Springman, my favorite sister, got me off the couch—at least for 10-ish miles a week.

Leroy and Belinda Kruse have patiently endured parenting me, the extent of which I have only been fully able to appreciate as a parent myself.

God put Jamie Sorensen in my path at just the right time. She introduced me to Trim Healthy Mama. I am in awe of her faith and steadfastness in circumstances the word frustration can't even begin to describe and her willingness to guide me in similar situations that pale in comparison.

The past, present, and future members of the Freshwater Wednesday morning women's Bible study group are my sisters in the faith and provide love, prayer, and friendship for the journey called life.

Glenn Haggerty provided writing advice and insight for getting this to at least resemble an actual book. It has been a pleasure to assist him in publishing his work, and I'm beyond grateful that he would invest in my efforts at passing along my experience in written form.

# About The Author

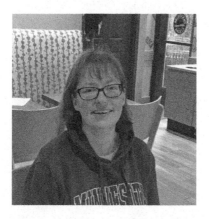

Carrie Carlson is not a writer and only blogs occasionally.
With a background in IT and PC support, she currently
homeschools her children and works as an all-purpose utility
person for a small publishing firm. Carrie holds a certificate
in pastoral leadership and spends her free time studying and
teaching Scripture, jogging, scrapbooking, knitting, and
reading. She lives in Minneapolis with her husband
and three daughters.

You can visit her blog at www.flowerkraut.com.

Made in the USA
Monee, IL
13 September 2020